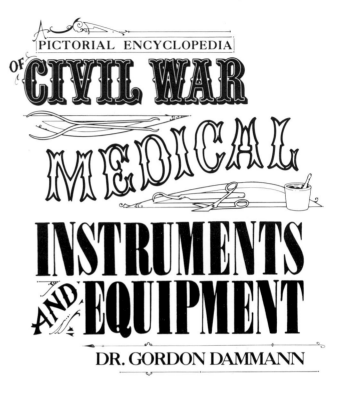

A PICTORIAL ENCYCLOPEDIA

CIVIL WAR MEDICAL INSTRUMENTS AND EQUIPMENT

DR. GORDON DAMMANN

VOLUME II

A PICTORIAL ENCYCLOPEDIA of CIVIL WAR MEDICAL INSTRUMENTS AND EQUIPMENT

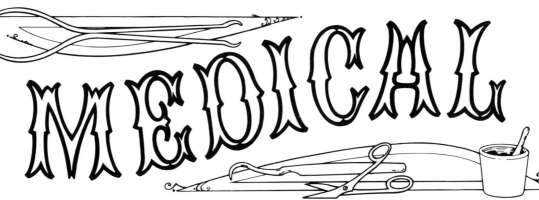

DR. GORDON DAMMANN

VOLUME II

PICTORIAL HISTORIES PUBLISHING COMPANY

Missoula, Montana 59801

LIBRARY OF CONGRESS
CATALOG CARD NUMBER 88-60472

ISBN 0-933126-94-8

First Printing: April 1988

Typography: Arrow Graphics, Missoula, Montana
Layout: Stan Cohen

PICTORIAL HISTORIES PUBLISHING COMPANY
713 South Third West
Missoula, Montana 59801

Contents

Acknowledgments

*I*f you asked me what gives me the most fun in the hobby of Civil War memorabilia collecting, I'd answer that it's the friends to be made. Since 1982, when Volume 1 of this book was finished, I've met many new people at places such as Ashland, Ohio; Gettysburg, Pa.; Wheaton, Ill.; and Richmond, Va. These are sites of some of the Civil War collectors' shows. We all set up and tear down our displays together and just have a good time.

The hours spent at places such as The Farnsworth House, Dobbins House and The Room Upstairs are worth the many hours of preparation and driving. One particular group is special to me—the battlefield tour group of the Chicago Civil War Round Table. If ever you want four days of great company and education, take the group's tour. There is nothing like it.

I'm reluctant to single out particular people who helped with this book for fear of leaving somebody out. I'll try, though.

Karen, Greg and Doug, you push when I need pushing and even tour Gettysburg with me at 6 a.m.

The Bradys of Kalamazoo and the Wheats of Virginia. Everybody should have friends such as these.

Mr. Peter D'onofrio and the "Society of Civil War Surgeons."

Alex and Susan Peck. Alex is rapidly becoming the expert on antique medical instruments.

Dr. and Mrs. James Dickson of Chambersburg and Dr. and Mrs. Sam Kirkpatrick of Hanover. They provide a home away from home in the Gettysburg area.

Mr. and Mrs. Don Williams of Ashland, Ohio; Dean Thomas of Gettysburg; "Hawkeye" Nowak of Wheaton and the Duggans of Richmond. If you want a successful Civil War show, look up these people.

Other friends: Dave Taylor, Jim Frasca, Bob Walters, Dan Weinberg, Marshall Krolick, Merle and Pat Sumner, Dr. Terry Hambrecht, Paul Milliken, Lewis Leigh and family, Paul DeHaan and family, Vick and Millie Vickery, Loren and Patty Golden, Dr. Audrey Davis of the Smithsonian, Dr. Richard Glenner, Seward Osborne, Marie Melchiori, the Cliojnacki brothers, Jack Magune and the Loyal Legion Library and Museum. All I can say is thank you, and may God bless you.

Finally, thanks, Jeri and Dr. Bob, for proofreading—again.

About the Author

*D*r. Gordon Dammann practices dentistry in Lena, Illinois. He has lectured throughout the country on the subject of Civil War medicine and his displays have won many awards. During the fall he officiates and coaches football on the junior high school, high school and college level. Greg and Doug are four years older and Karen refuses to talk about it.

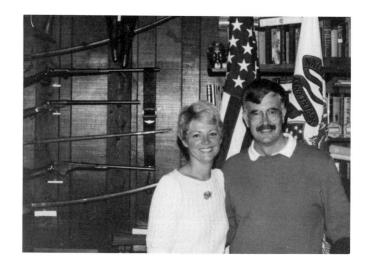

Faces of Surgeons

Since the subject of this book is the Medical Service or Department during the Civil War, it is appropriate that we begin with the men who were responsible for medical care—the surgeons and the assistant surgeons. Look at their faces. Study them. Imagine what must have been on their minds when these photos were taken. Look to the picture and documents of Surgeon R.R. McMeens of Ohio. Here is a man who gave his life for the medical care of his men. He could have left the service and gone home to his loving wife in Sandusky, Ohio; however, he stayed with his men. On October 15, 1862, he suffered a heart attack and was listed as a medical casualty of the Civil War.

Most historians do not try to discover the inner thoughts of the people they write about, but I have done this with Surgeon McMeens. He was a loving husband and a man of great patriotic feelings for his country. He felt that his men needed him, and in a way he needed them. Had he returned home he might have lived a few more years with thoughts that would have "nagged" at his soul. As it was, he died a true patriot. That is the way he wanted his life to end. This book is dedicated to all the Surgeon McMeenses of both the Union and Confederate armies. They did not die in vain.

Personal letters from Surgeon McMeens and his friends reveal much about the man who was born in Lycoming County, Pennsylvania, on February 26, 1820. He was graduated from the University of Pennsylvania School of Medicine in 1841. In 1843 he married Ann C. Pettenger, and in 1846 they moved to Sandusky, Ohio.

His friend, a Dr. Shumard, wrote to Governor Tod after McMeens' death: "It is with feelings of deepest regret that I have to announce the death of Surgeon R.R. McMeens of the 3rd Regt. Ohio Vol. Army, which occurred suddenly at Perryville, Kentucky. Surgeon McMeens was among the first to offer his services to this country after the breaking out of the rebellion.

"Entering the three-months service as a regimental surgeon, McMeens immediately was ordered to Camp Dennison, where his gentlemanly deportment and great professional skill soon won for him the esteem and confidence of his brother officers, at whose request he was appointed medical director of the post. All the arduous duties of which office he performed in such a manner as to win for him the warmest commendations of the Surgeon General of the State.

"From that time until the period of his death, he has continued in actual service, filling many important positions in the Medical Department of the Army.

"Shortly before the Battle of Perryville, he was appointed medical director to the troops under the command of the lamented Jackson, and after having participated actively in the battle, was detailed to assist in taking care of the wounded at Perryville, in which position his kindness of heart, sound judgment and great professional skill enabled him to contribute very largely toward the relief of our suffering soldiers.

"He has fallen while nobly working at his post; although suffering greatly from disease, he refused to abandon his work and performed several important surgical operations only a few hours before his death."

Surgeon McMeens was not the only man to distinguish himself during the Civil War. Many more healing professionals, both Northern and Southern, saw their duty and met the challenge.

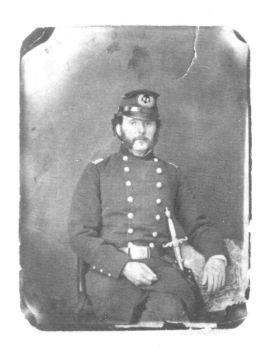

Surgeon R.R. McMeens, 1820-1862.

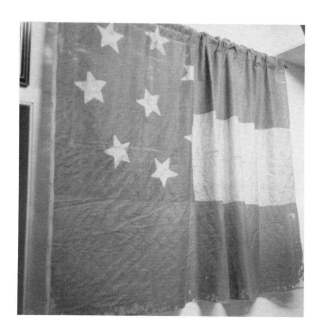

Captured Confederate flag sent home to Ohio by Surgeon McMeens.

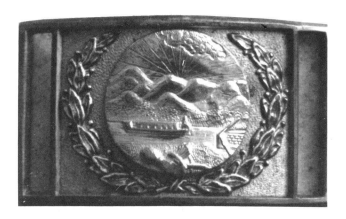

State of Ohio belt buckle that belonged to Surgeon McMeens.

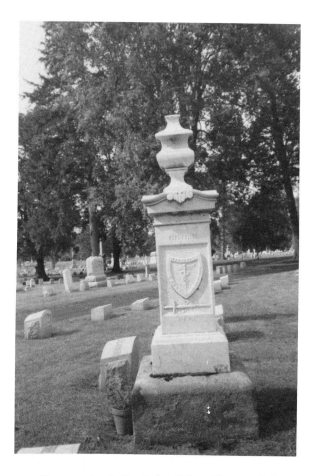

Grave marker in Sandusky, Ohio, of Surgeon R.R. McMeens and Mrs. McMeens.

Surgeon John Wiley was born on August 7, 1815, near Penns Grove, New Jersey. His father, David, was a prosperous farmer, and John attended Jefferson Medical College for three full academic years. After his graduation in 1837, he practiced medicine in Cape May Court House, New Jersey. On December 23, 1845, he married Daniela Hand. They had three children, although their son died in infancy.

With the outbreak of the Civil War in 1861, John had reached the age of 46. His wife was a semi-invalid; therefore, he had many responsibilities to weigh before entering the service of his country. After Bull Run, he offered his service and was commissioned surgeon of the 6th New Jersey Volunteer Infantry on August 17, 1861. He served with distinction as regimental surgeon, then as surgeon-in-chief, 3rd Brigade, 2nd Division, 3rd Army Corps. On two occasions his horse was shot from under him, and he was favorably mentioned in the battle reports of Second Bull Run and Chancellorsville.

His record reads like a roll-call of the Army of the Potomac: Siege of Yorktown, Williamsburg, Fair Oaks and Seven Pines, Savage's Station, Glendale, Malvern Hill, Second Bull Run, Chantilly, Centreville, Fredericksburg, Chancellorsville, Gettysburg, Mine Run, Wilderness, Cold Harbor, Petersburg Siege, Deep Bottom Run, the Battle of the Crater and North Bank of James River. He was captured and held for 10 days after Second Bull Run. He was offered the post of division surgeon, but felt that his wife's illness required a return home. He was mustered out on September 7, 1864. His wife died in 1873, and he remarried in 1877. Dr. Wiley died on December 24, 1891, and his resting place is the Baptist Cemetery in Cape May Court House.

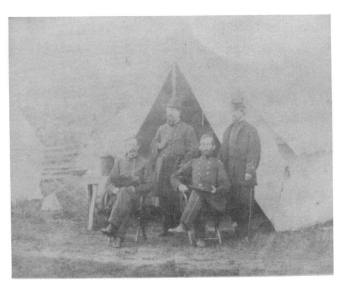

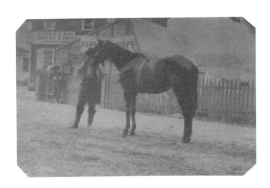

Tintype of Surgeon Wiley's horse.

Surgeon Wiley is the officer seated at the right. This albumen was taken in front of his tent in 1862.

CDV of Surgeon Wiley's wife and daughter at the time of the Civil War.

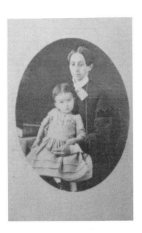

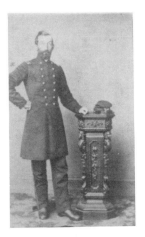

CDV of Surgeon John A. Wiley, 6th New Jersey Volunteer Infantry.

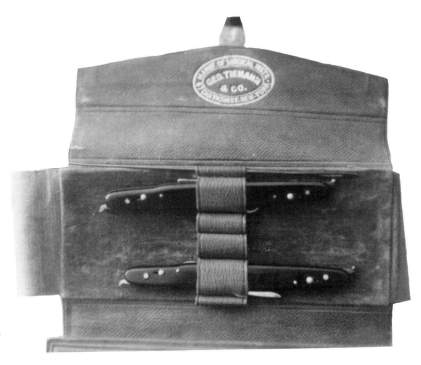

Surgeon Wiley's pocket kit, manufactured by Tiemann's.

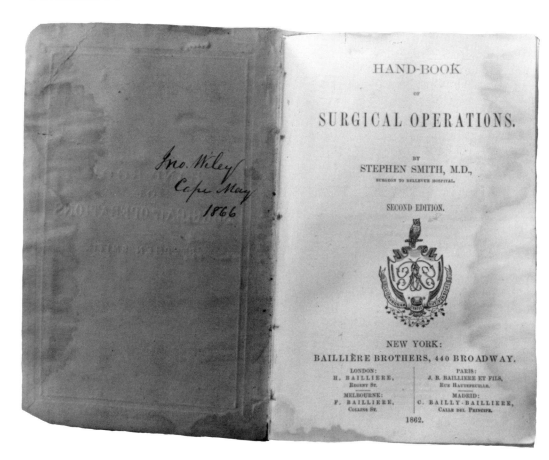

Surgeon Wiley's handbook.

Medical officer's sword that belonged to Surgeon Horace Potter of the 105th Illinois Volunteer Infantry. Surgeon Potter lost his life while looking for a site for his hospital on June 2, 1864, near Kingston, Georgia.

Surgeon Potter's grave stone, which contains the artillery shell that took his life.

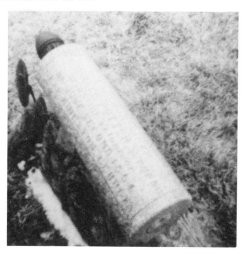

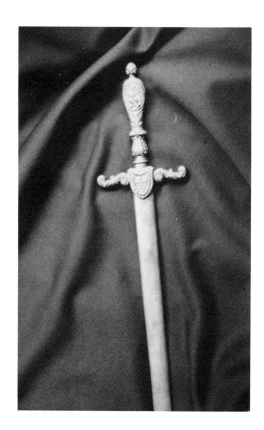

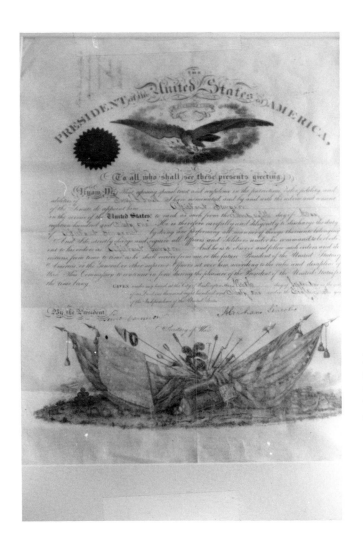

Military commission signed by President Lincoln. This commission was given to Assistant Surgeon Joseph S. Smith on September 9, 1861. Surgeon Smith served throughout the War and died fighting a yellow fever epidemic in 1867 at Fort Jefferson, Dry Tortugas.

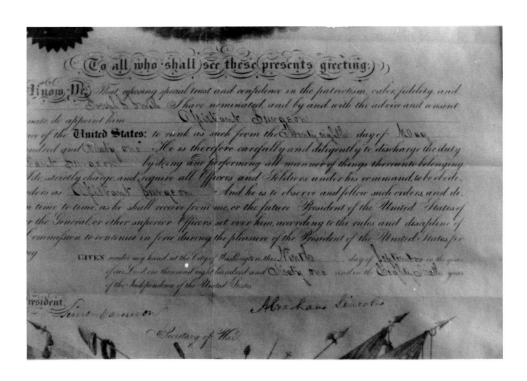

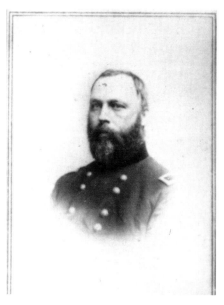

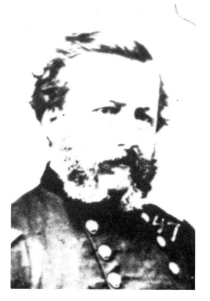

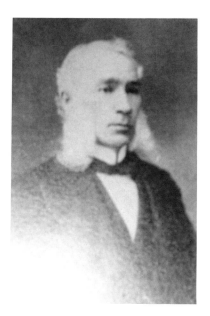

CDV and autograph of Surgeon General William A. Hammond. Hammond served from 1861-1864. He is the father of the Army Medical Corps.

Surgeon General Joseph Barnes. Surgeon General from 1864-1882. He attended to President Lincoln the night of the assassination and the morning after.

Surgeon General Samuel Moore, C.S.A. He served the Confederate States as head of its medical department for the duration of the war.

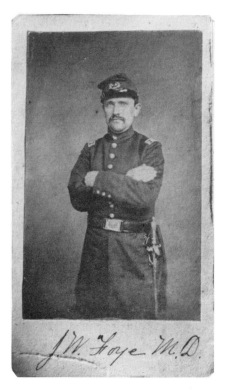

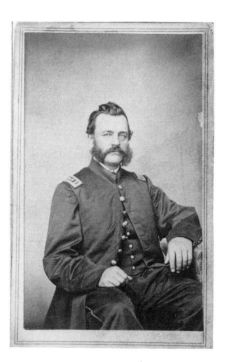

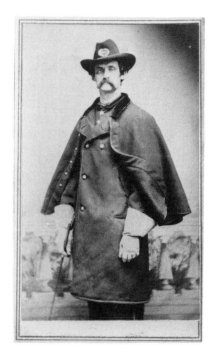

Surgeon Dunean. The MS shoulder straps are very distinctive.

Unidentified surgeon with distinctive officer's cape and gauntlets.

John W. Foye, assistant surgeon, 11th M.V.I. Notice the surgeon's bummers cap, shoulder straps, belt buckle and sword.

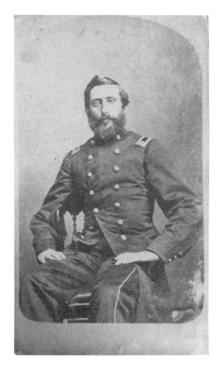

Surgeon J.R. Zearing of the 57th Illinois Volunteer Infantry. He is wearing a double-breasted coat and major's shoulder straps.

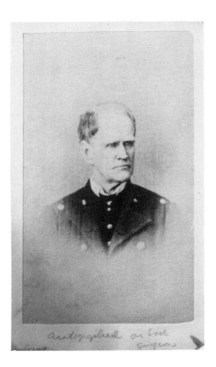

Surgeon George W. Stipp, medical inspector, U.S. Army. Notice the different coat and oak leaves on the shoulders.

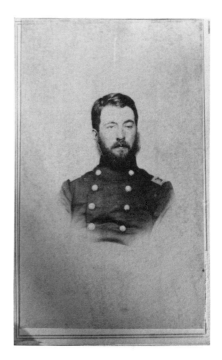

Surgeon Joseph E. Murta of the 8th Wisconsin Infantry.

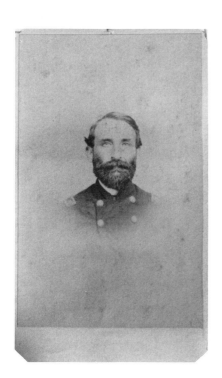

Surgeon Rohrer of the 10th Pennsylvania Reserves.

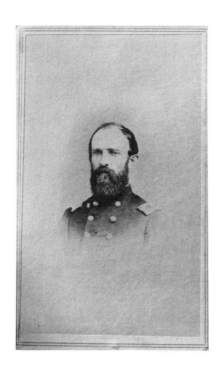

Surgeon Theodore S. Christ of the 45th Pennsylvania Volunteers.

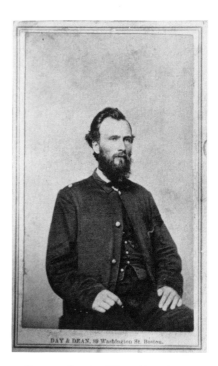

Surgeon Snyder. His uniform is devoid of insignia except for what looks like a major's leaf on the right shoulder.

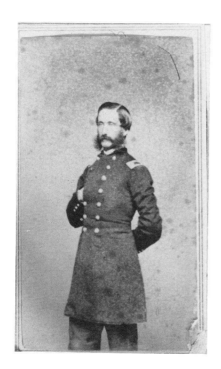

Surgeon Edwin McDonald, medical director of the District of Baton Rouge.

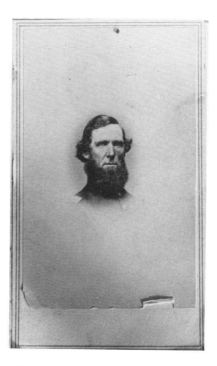

Surgeon George F. Thompson, assistant surgeon of the 38th Mass.

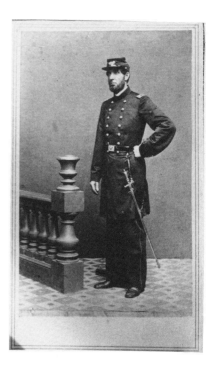

Standing pose of a surgeon wearing Kepie, coat, pants, sword belt and sword.

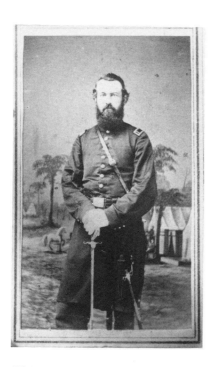

This front view shows a cross belt of the sword belt.

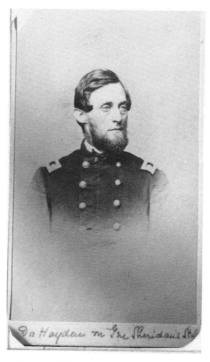

Surgeon Haydan was a member of General Sheridan's staff.

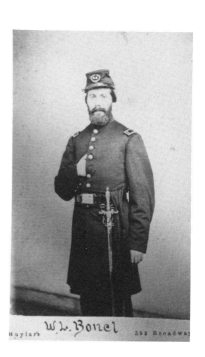

Surgeon W.L. Bonel, assistant surgeon of the 53rd Regiment. This full-face view shows the hat insignia, sash, sword belt and sword.

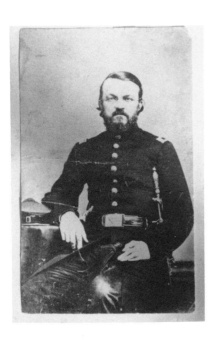

Surgeon Siefert of the 38th Mass.

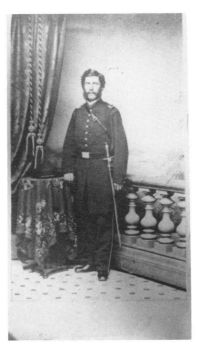

Assistant Surgeon W.B. Chambers of the 60th New York.

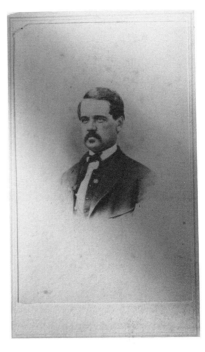

Surgeon, Hobell General Hospital, Portsmouth Grove, Rhode Island.

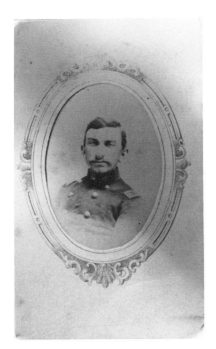

Surgeon Henry Martin.

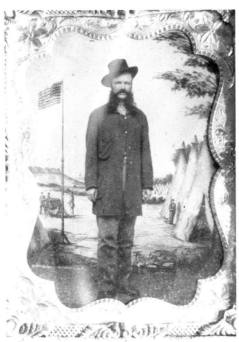

Surgeon William Nichols Jr. of the 2nd Massachusetts Infantry. Notice his very non-regulation uniform, which is devoid of any insignia. It looks like an enlisted man's uniform.

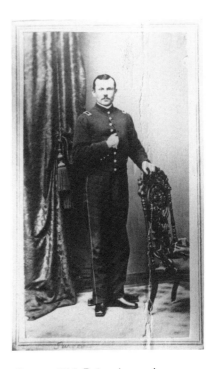

Surgeon J.M. Bohemien, acting surgeon, U.S. Army. This is a rare view of a surgeon in a short coat. He might have been attached to a cavalry regiment.

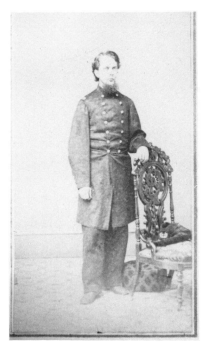

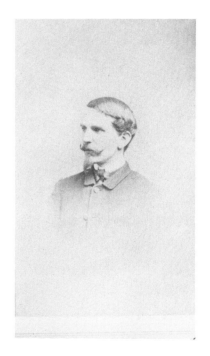

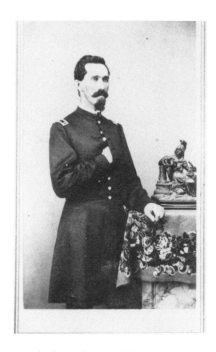

An unidentified surgeon. A nice example of an officer's slouch hat is on the chair.

CDV of Surgeon McClellan, who was an assistant medical director for the Army.

Assistant Surgeon Huntington.

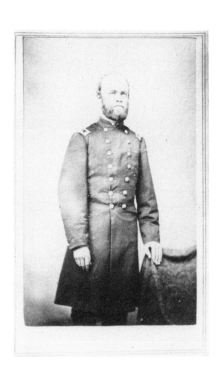

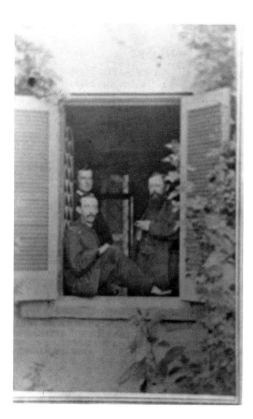

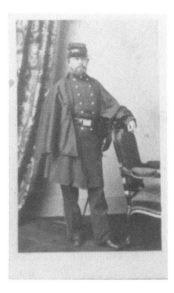

CDV of Surgeon Bontecou. He photographed all wounded Union soldiers for the purpose of keeping records. There is believed to be more than 2,000 of these photographs.

Surgeon Absalom B. Steward of the 1st Alabama (Union) Cavalry. Mustered into the army on 7-8-1863 and mustered out on 1-23-1864.

CDV of Surgeon Bontecou. He is seated on the left in this window at Fort Monroe.

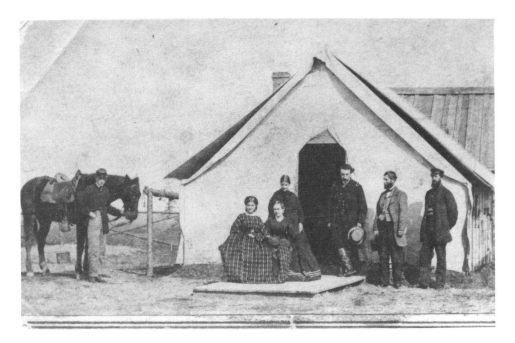

Surgeon King of the Pennsylvania Volunteer Infantry. Positioned in front of a large hospital tent are Surgeon King, Mrs. King and his hospital steward. The horse belonged to Surgeon King.

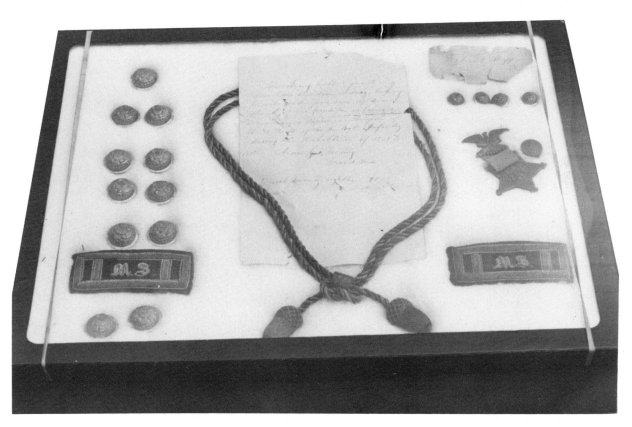

In Volume I, Illustration No. 161 shows a grouping of surgeon's insignia that belonged to a surgeon of the 78th Pennsylvania Volunteer Infantry. The note states that "Grandma gives these relics to grandson, Sidney, so that he will remember Grandpa as a surgeon who served through the War." With the help of Marie Melchiori and the records of the 78th, it was discovered that three surgeons had served through the War and only one had a grandson named Sidney. These items belonged to Surgeon Florilla Morris.

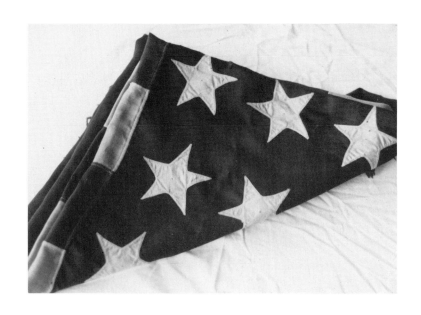

A 36-star U.S. flag brought back from the War by Surgeon Jacob R. Weist of the 1st U.S.C.T. Surgeon Weist was from Richmond, Indiana, and in his notes he states that this flag flew over Atlanta, Georgia, at one time. The flag measures 60 inches by 72 inches.

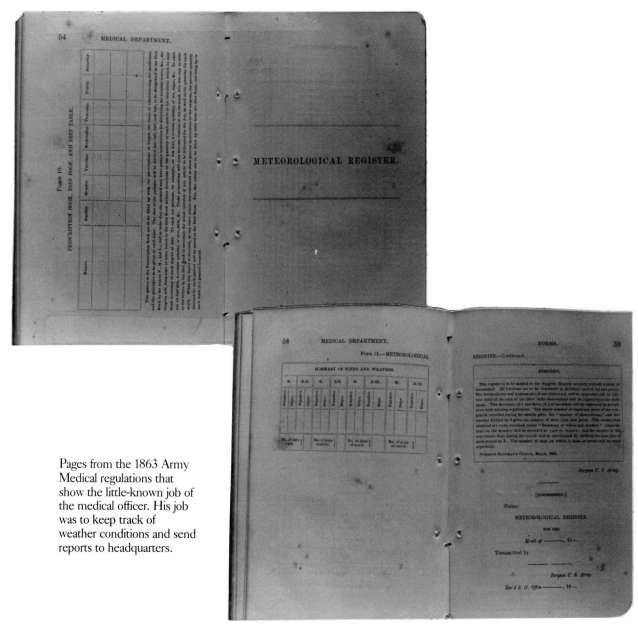

Pages from the 1863 Army Medical regulations that show the little-known job of the medical officer. His job was to keep track of weather conditions and send reports to headquarters.

The Wounded Veteran

"*T*he Empty Sleeve" was a term that had great impact on the population during and after the Civil War. It signifies the way most wounded veterans returned home —with an empty sleeve or trouser leg. If the soldier did not pay with his life, most likely he paid with the loss of one or more limbs. Gunshot or shrapnel wounds that involved the major blood vessels or large bones of the region necessitated amputation. This was the accepted medical treatment for this kind of trauma. It can be verified in any medical textbook of the 1850s and 1860s.

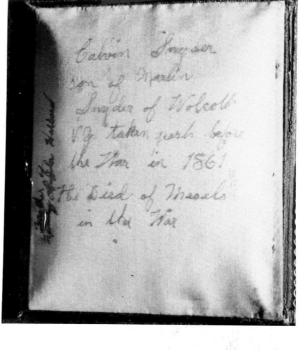

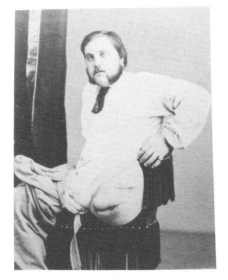

Illustration of a soldier with an amputation of the leg at the hip joint. 1st Sgt. Ulmer (15th N.J. Vol.) was fortunate to have survived because more than 89 percent of the patients with this type of surgery died.

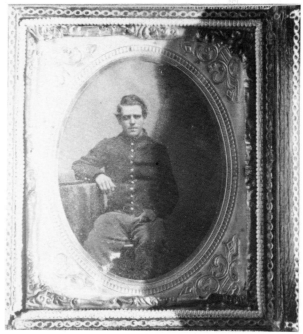

Calvin Snyder—The inscription alongside his tintype tells that he died of the simple disease of measles, as did more than 3,215 others. He was 18 when he died.

Soldiers with various amputations.

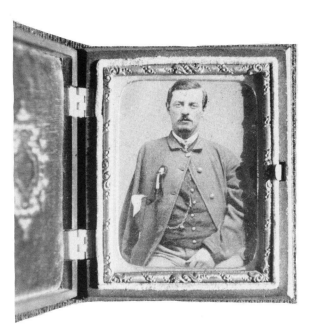

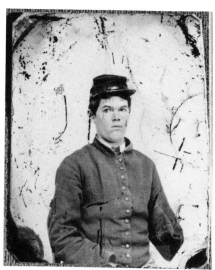

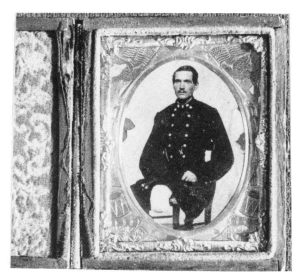

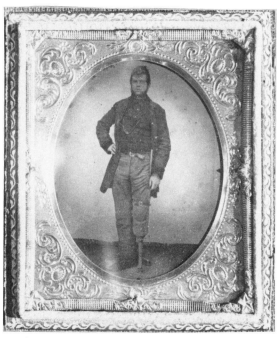

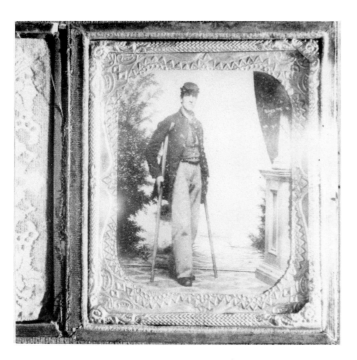

Tintype of a soldier using crutches.

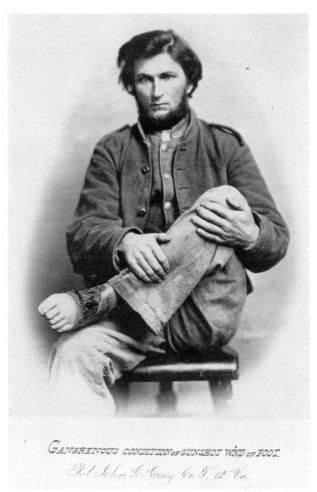

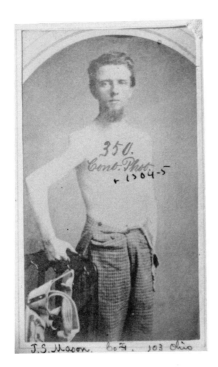

J.S. Mason of the 103rd Ohio. This photo shows the effect of a resection operation of the shoulder and upper arm area. Notice the splint device on the chair. It helped support the arm. This photo was probably one of Bontecou's.

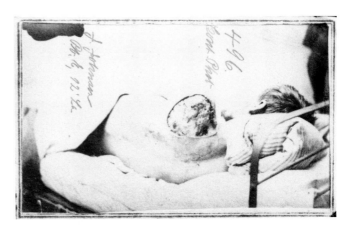

Jacob Johnson of the 12th Louisiana Volunteer Infantry. The photo of a Confederate soldier was taken at Hospital 1, Nashville, Tennessee. The wound is a fractured scapula and resulting loss of soft tissue.

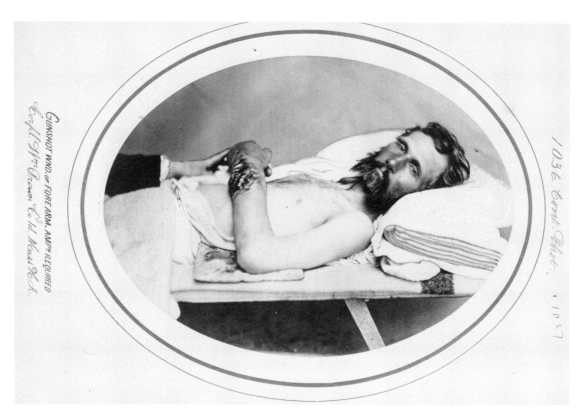

Courtesy of Armed Forces Institute of Pathology, Walter Reed Army Hospital.

Mortal wound of the upper leg. This probably is a post-mortem photo because the man is wearing a chin-strap. Courtesy of Armed Forces Institute of Pathology, Walter Reed Army Hospital.

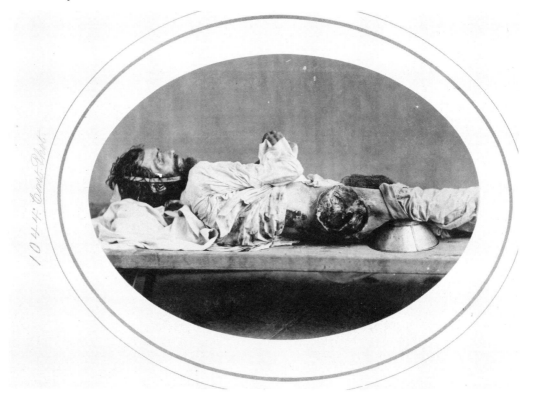

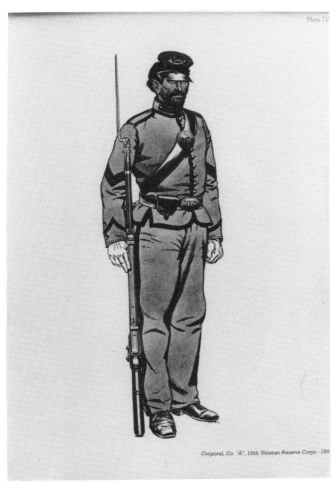

Corporal, Co. 'A', 10th Veteran Reserve Corps—186

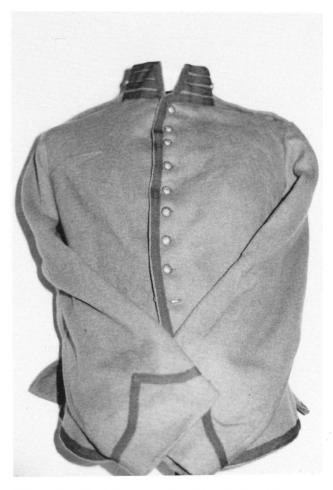

Distinctive waist jacket worn by members of the "Invalid Corps." The color of the jacket is sky blue with dark blue piping and shoulder strap edges. There are 12 enlisted eagle buttons on the front of the jacket. The Invalid Veterans Reserve Corp was made up of wounded soldiers who could perform some camp duty, mostly guard duty.

VETERANS RESERVE CORPS or INVALID CORPS

Tintype of a member of the Veterans Reserve Corps, or "Invalid Corps."

Certificate of enlistment into the Invalid Corps signed by a surgeon.

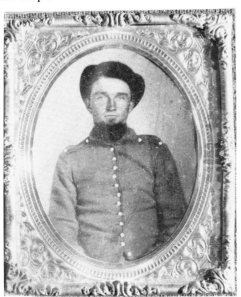

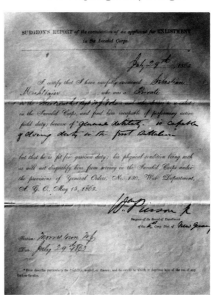

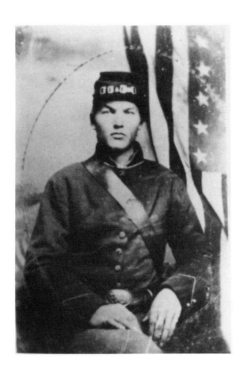

Peleg Bradford of the 1st Maine Heavy Artillery was wounded on June 17, 1864, at the Siege of Petersburg.

One of Peleg Bradford's artificial legs that he wore after his discharge. Peleg survived two amputations. He returned to Maine, where he fathered eight children and lived until 1921.

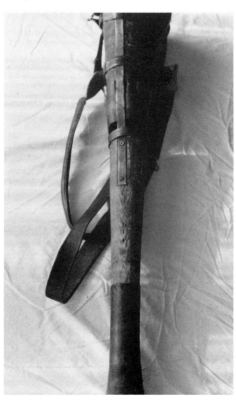

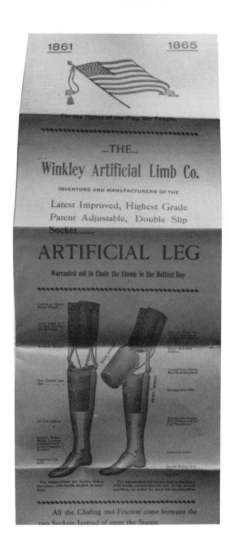

Documents used by Peleg Bradford to obtain a prosthetic leg. The U.S. government paid a certain amount to each veteran to have an artificial device constructed. The advertisement shows the type of artificial leg made for Peleg Bradford in Minneapolis, Minnesota.

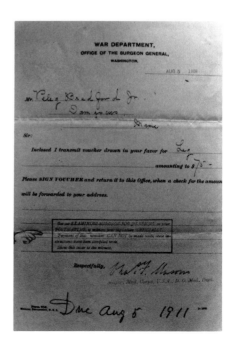

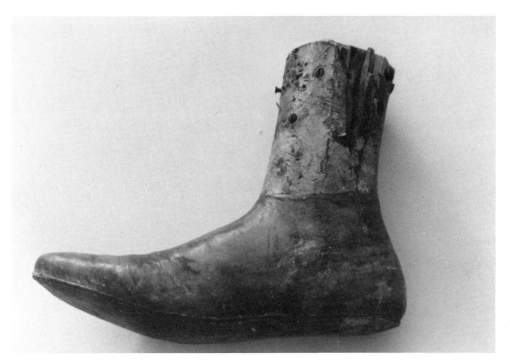

Prosthetic or wooden foot used by an amputee after the Civil War. Many different devices were constructed to aid the wounded veteran. Many types of artificial arms and legs were patented during the late 1860s and 1870s.

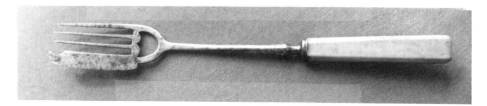

Amputee's combination knife and fork, which was very common during and after the Civil War.

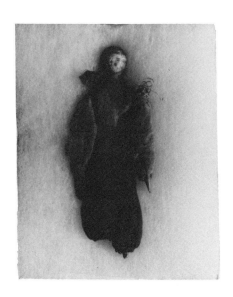

"Clothespin dolls" were sold by some veterans in order to help support themselves. These were constructed from a wooden clothespin and were attired in patriotic colors. Sometimes the material came from uniforms or pieces of battleflags. Most dolls depicted the wound of the veteran. In this particular case the doll had an amputated right leg.

Hospitals of the Civil War

*W*ith the beginning of the Civil War in 1861, both armies were faced with the fact that they were ill-prepared for the wounded soldier and what to do with him. At the beginning of the War, there was not one military hospital in the country. The only post hospital was at Fort Leavenworth, Kansas, and it had 40 beds. After the first Battle of Bull Run, Washington, D.C., was overrun with wounded. Every public building was used as a hospital—even the Capitol.

Surgeon William A. Hammond oversaw the building of general hospitals for the Union. By 1863 there were more than 151 hospitals; by the War's end there were 204 with a bed capacity of 136,894. Washington had more than 16 general hospitals; others were located in Philadelphia (Satterlee General, with 3,500 beds), New York, Baltimore, Chattanooga, Louisville, Memphis, Nashville, City Point in Virginia, and Jefferson, Indiana. These hospitals made up the Union general-hospital system.

The Confederacy had about 150 general hospitals. The largest, Chimborazo, had 8,000 beds and was in Richmond.

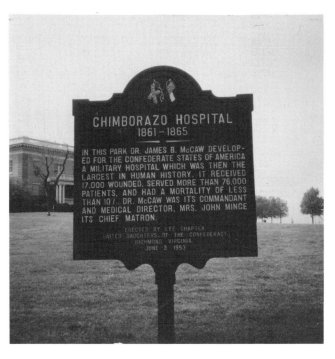

The largest general hospital of the Civil War was Chimborazo. Located in Richmond, it had a bed capacity of 8,000. The complex was situated on a bluff overlooking the city and fresh breezes provided good ventilation. Surgeon McGaw developed a hospital vegetable garden and a herd of beef and dairy cattle to feed his patients.

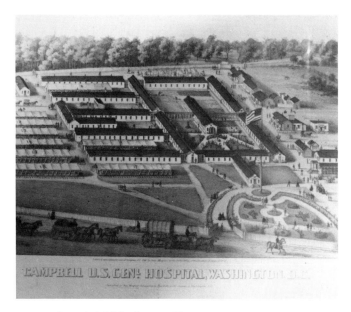

Campbell U.S. General Hospital was one of 16 general hospitals in Washington, D.C. It had a bed capacity of 1,600. As can be seen in the lithograph, hospitals were designed in the "pavilion plan." Each ward was self-contained off of a central hub. This allowed for ventilation and gave the ability to seal off a ward if necessary.

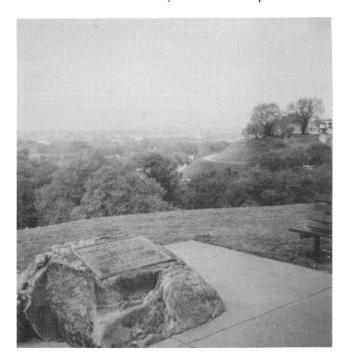

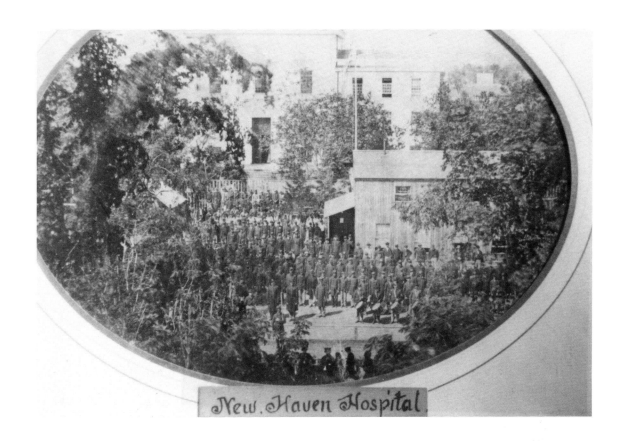

Typical of general hospitals in large cities, New Haven Hospital (above) and Nashville (below) accommodated many wounded and sick soldiers.

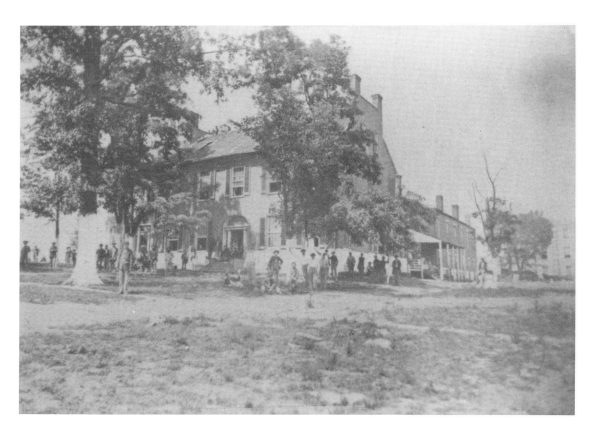

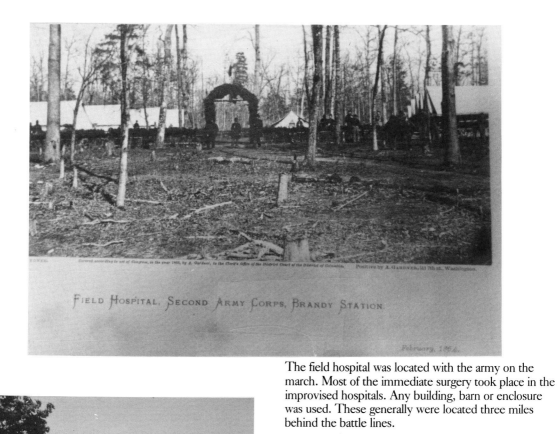

FIELD HOSPITAL, SECOND ARMY CORPS, BRANDY STATION.

February, 1864.

The field hospital was located with the army on the march. Most of the immediate surgery took place in the improvised hospitals. Any building, barn or enclosure was used. These generally were located three miles behind the battle lines.

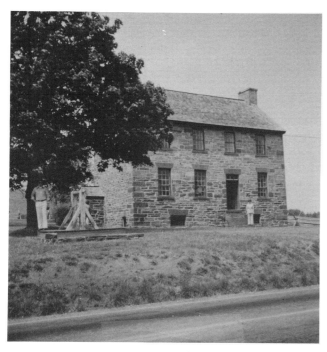

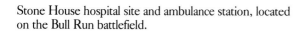

Stone House hospital site and ambulance station, located on the Bull Run battlefield.

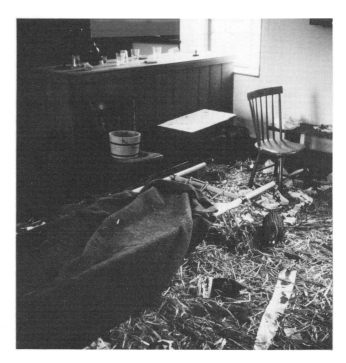

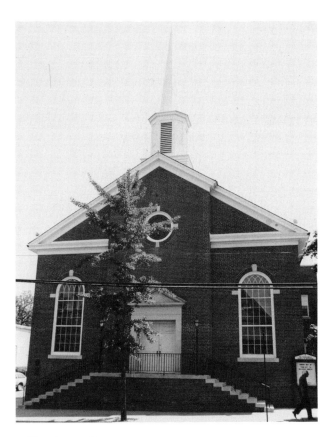

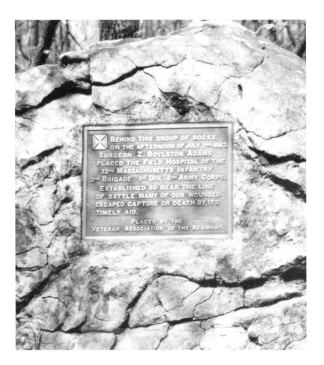

Churches at Gettysburg were used as field hospitals. Just about every building in Gettysburg was turned into a resting place for wounded soldiers.

The only monument to a field dressing station is located on the Gettysburg battlefield. At dressing stations, wounds were treated immediately. Able men were sent back to battle and severely wounded men were transported by stretcher or ambulance to the field hospital.

Field hospital as shown on the Gettysburg Cyclorama.

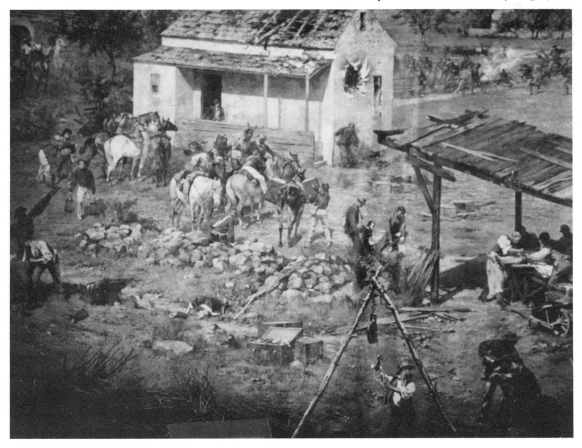

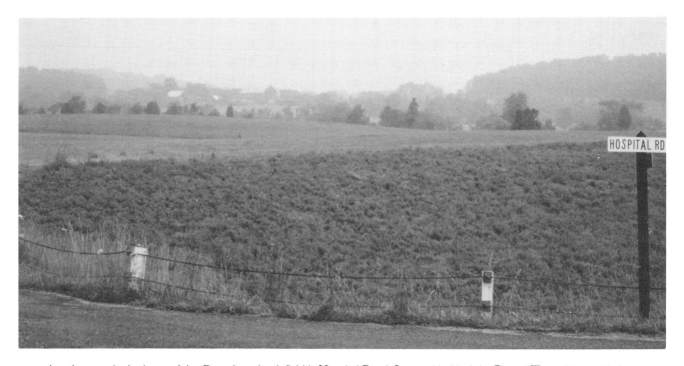

An often overlooked part of the Gettysburg battlefield is Hospital Road. Located behind the Round Tops, this road led to most of the corps hospitals. Most of the original buildings are still present, but they are private property and should be respected as such. There are markers at each site. Also, through the efforts of historians on staff at Gettysburg National Battlefield, many hospital sites are identified with distinctive blue signs.

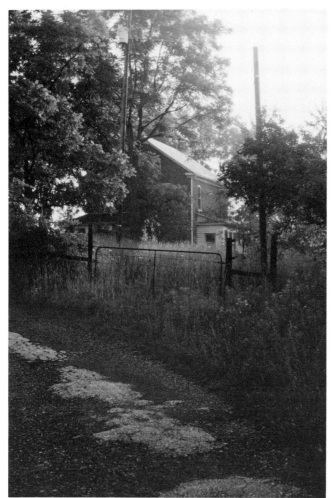

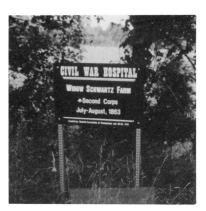

The Schwartz farm buildings housed the Third Corps hospitals, not the Second.

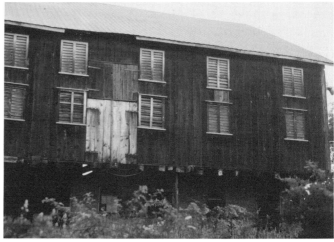

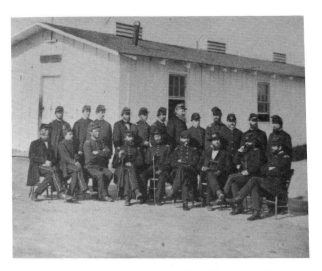

Staff surgeons in front of an unidentified hospital.

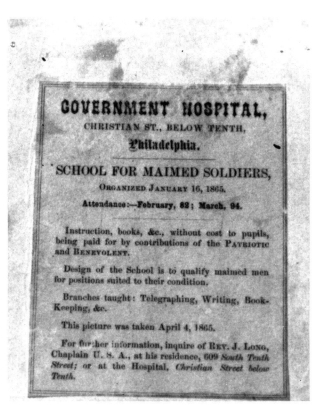

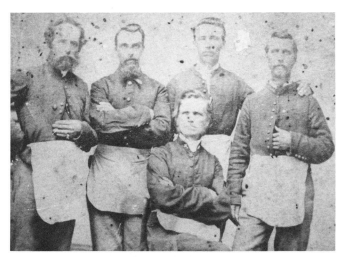

Hospital attendants with a staff chaplain.

The "Lincoln Institute" took maimed soldiers and tried to train them for possible employment. This hospital taught telegraphing, writing and bookkeeping. This was the beginning of veterans hospitals.

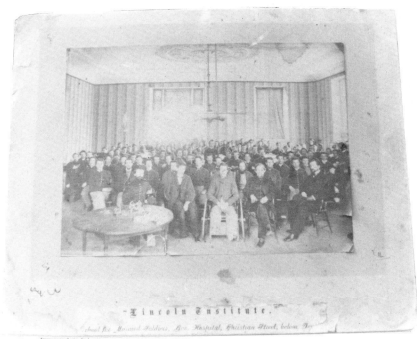

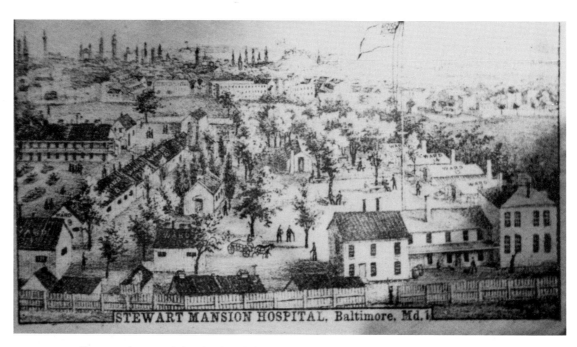

One popular way of showing hospitals was in the form of envelopes used by patients.

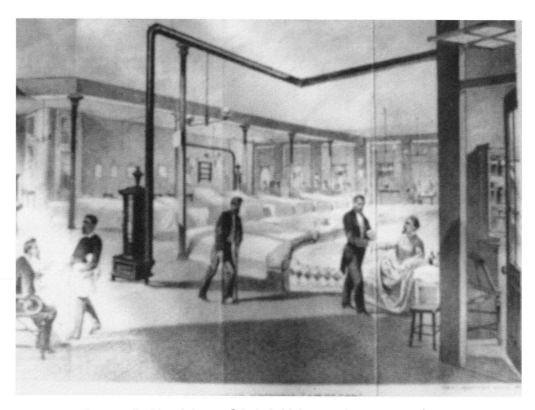

A very stylized hospital scene. It is doubtful that attendants wore tuxedos.

The following is a grouping of documents that came from some general Union hospitals.

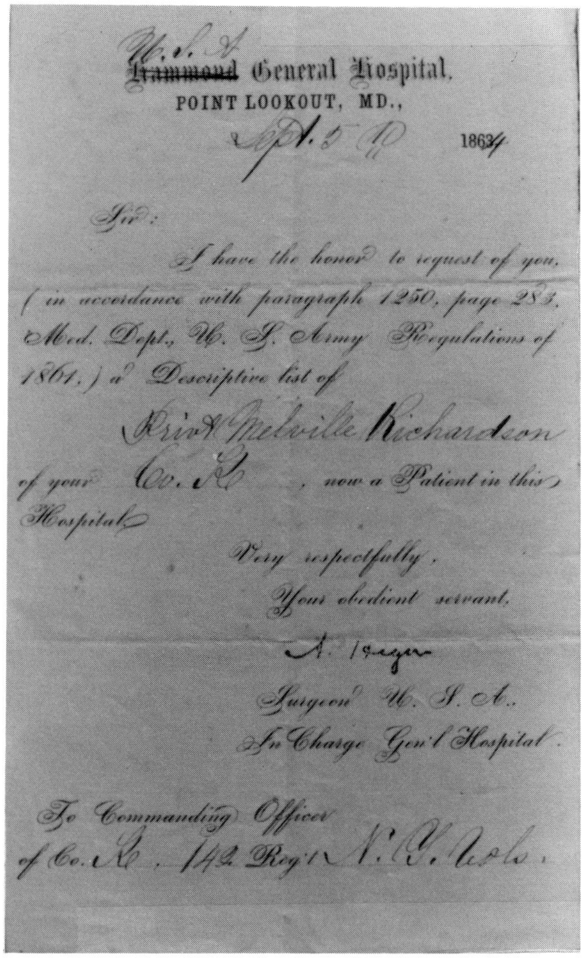
U. S. A. ~~Hammond~~ General Hospital,
POINT LOOKOUT, MD.,

Sept. 5 th 1864

Sir:

I have the honor to request of you, (in accordance with paragraph 1250, page 283, Med. Dept., U. S. Army Regulations of 1861,) a Descriptive list of

Privt Melville Richardson

of your Co. K, now a Patient in this Hospital.

Very respectfully,
Your obedient servant,
A. Heger
Surgeon U. S. A.
In Charge Gen'l Hospital.

To Commanding Officer
of Co. K, 142 Reg't N. Y. Vols.

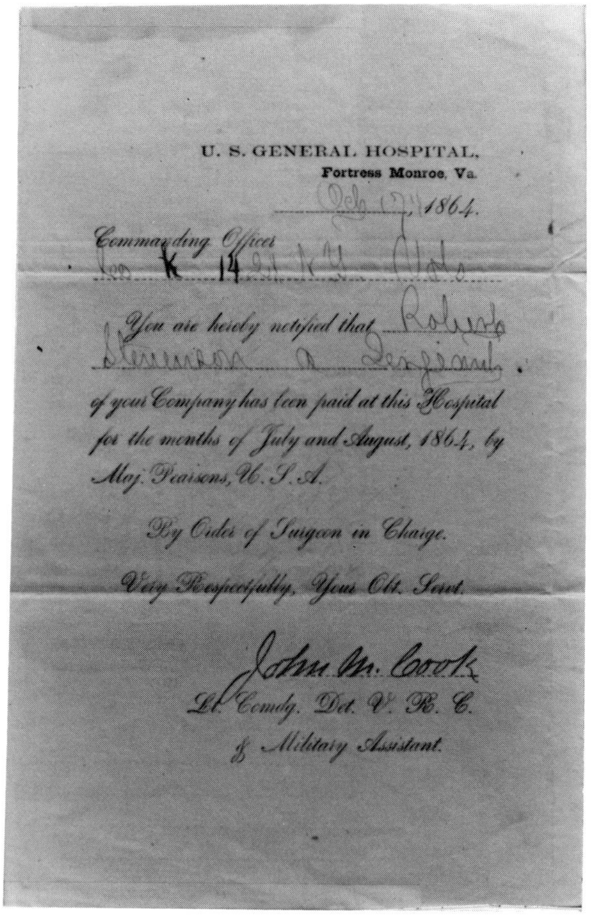
U. S. GENERAL HOSPITAL,
Fortress Monroe, Va.
Oct 17 1864.

Commanding Officer
Co K 142 N. Y. Vols.

You are hereby notified that Robert Stevenson a Sergeant of your Company has been paid at this Hospital for the months of July and August, 1864, by Maj. Pearsons, U. S. A.

By Order of Surgeon in Charge.

Very Respectfully, Your Obt. Servt.

John M. Cook
Lt. Comdg. Det. V. R. C.
& Military Assistant.

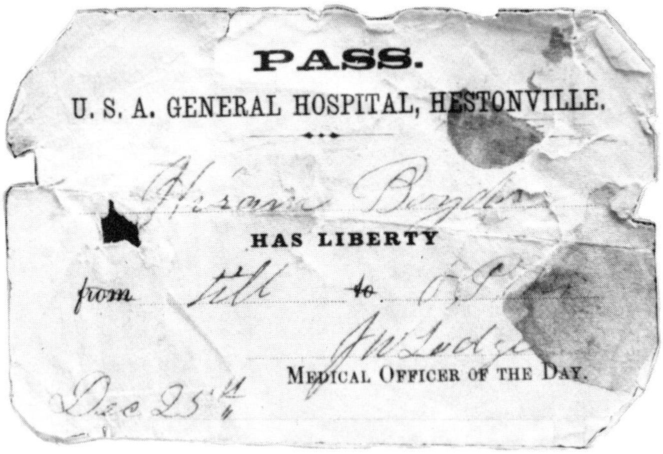
PASS.
U. S. A. GENERAL HOSPITAL, HESTONVILLE.

Hiram Boyden
HAS LIBERTY
from till to 6 P.M.
J W Lodge
MEDICAL OFFICER OF THE DAY.
Dec 25th 64

A hospital pass for the Hestonville Hospital dated December 25.

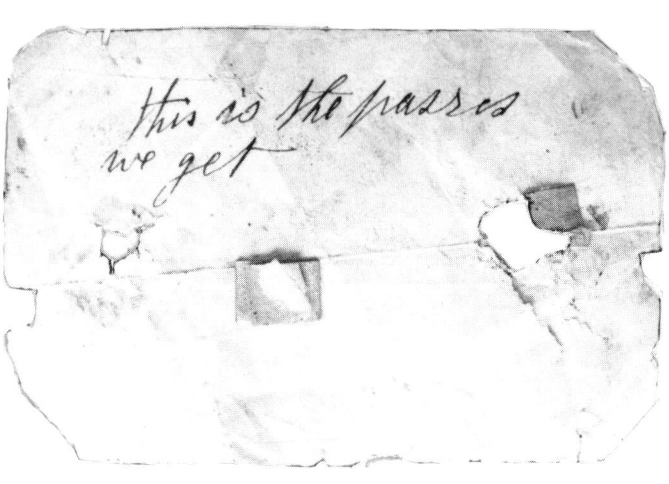
this is the passes
we get

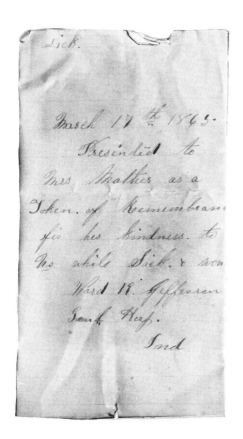

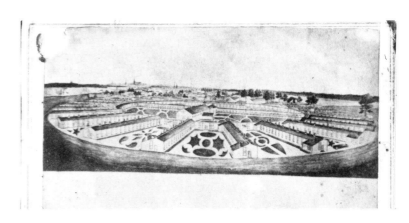

Jefferson, Indiana, General Hospital.

A note from a ward book of Jefferson General Hospital.

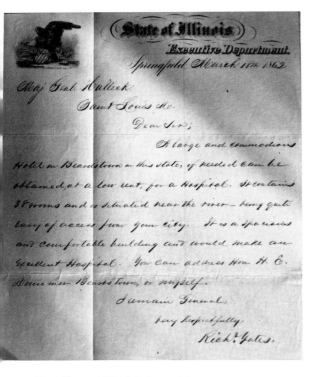

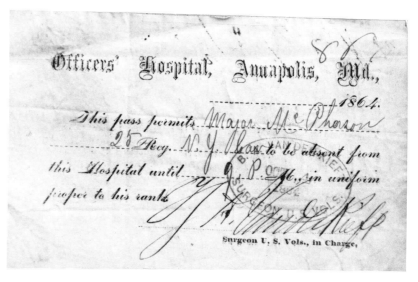

A pass issued to a patient so that he could visit friends outside the hospital.

Gov. Yates of Illinois informs Maj. Gen. Halleck by letter that a hotel in Beardstown, Illinois, can be requisitioned for a hospital.

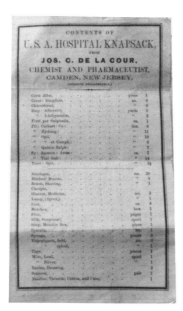

The following illustrations show the contents of the knapsack for hospital use dispensed by Jos. C. De La Cour of Camden, New Jersey.

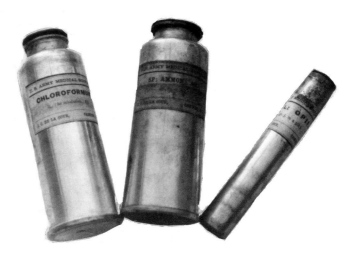

Metal medicine containers with screw tops. These were found to be stronger than glass and were used in the knapsack.

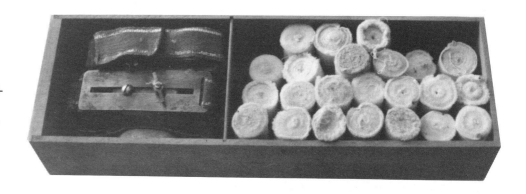

Drawer containing a tourniquet and bandage rolls for the De La Cour knapsack.

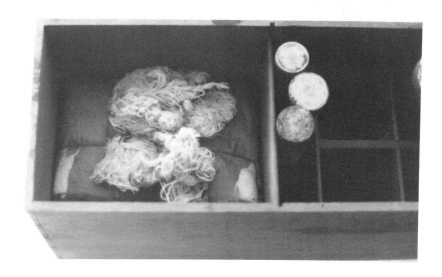

Absorbent lint from the De La Cour knapsack.

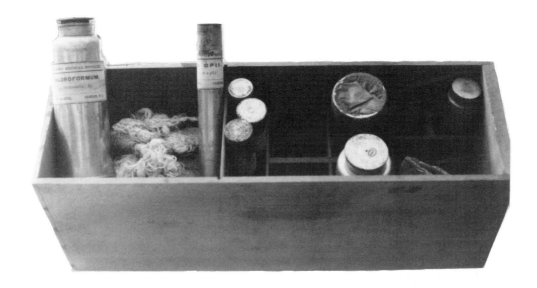

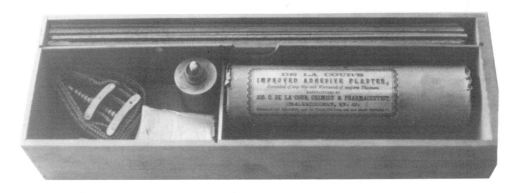

Shelf containing tourniquet, brass alcohol burner, splint material and adhesive plaster from the De La Cour knapsack.

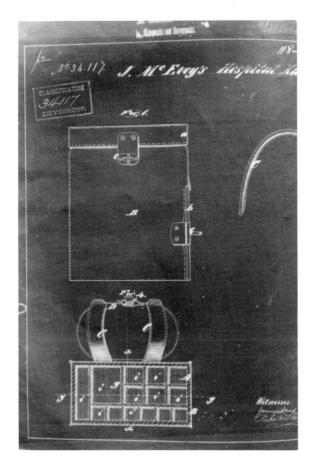

A copy of the original patent description for the McEvey's Hospital knapsack dated 1862.

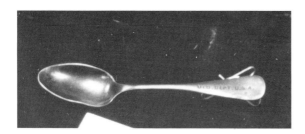

Pewter hospital department spoon.

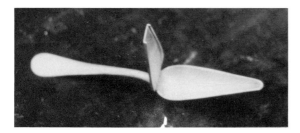

Pewter hospital department covered spoon for use by invalid.

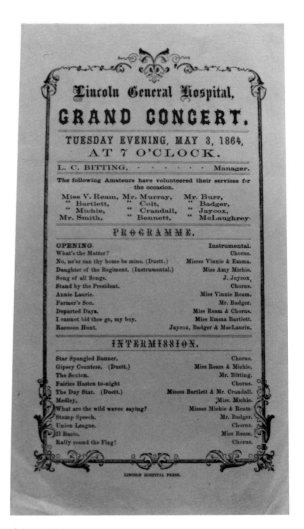

A broadside advertising a concert that would be given at Lincoln General Hospital on May 3, 1864.

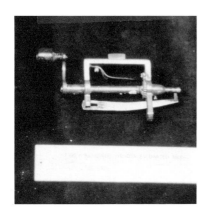

Bandage roller and cutter from the 1840-1860 era.

Porcelain invalid feeding spoons (handles are missing).

Porcelain invalid feeding cup.

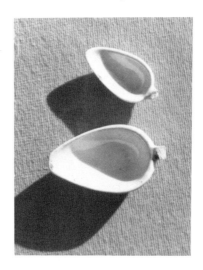

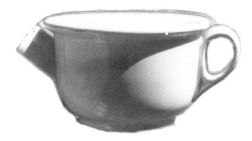

Nurses of the Civil War

*W*ith the advent of large general hospitals came the need for personnel to care for patients. Men who were able were needed on the line of battle, so the opportunity to serve fell to a new group of individuals, the women of America.

Moved by an indomitable desire to serve the victims of wounds and sickness in person, 3,200 women made their way to the bedsides of the sick and wounded men. They were impelled by instincts that assured them of their ability to endure hardships, overcome obstacles and adapt themselves to the unusual and unfeminine circumstances in which they were placed. Many women left their homes and children, risked their lives in fevered hospitals, lived in tents or hospital wagons, and incurred the unknowing gossip from home. They did all this for $12 a month and food.

Nursing was only part of their great devotion. Some worked with the Relief Commission in distributing needed items for the soldier's comfort. Others helped establish soldiers' homes or temporary soldiers' lodges to house those veterans in transit home or back to their units. Still others lent their support by scraping cloth into lint, knitting socks or sweaters, or baking the extras that soldiers looked forward to.

All in all, women's work in the Civil War was never-ending and always needed.

The following two pages contain CDVs of women who served as nurses during the Civil War. The two that are grouped together were found in a diary that deals with Jefferson, Indiana, General Hospital.

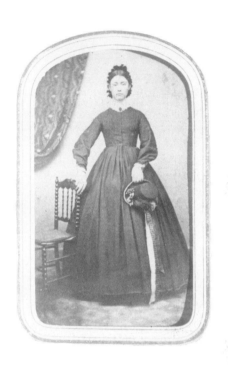

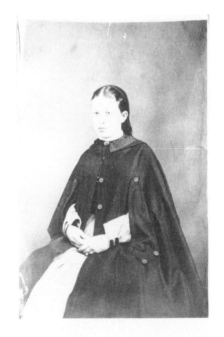

CDV of a nurse wearing a distinctive cape. As dictated by Dorthea Dix (head of the Union Nurse Corps), women should be plain-looking and be over the age of 30. Their clothes had to be of gray or black material that buttoned at the neck and extended to the floor.

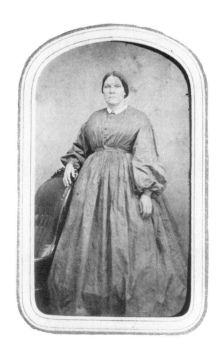

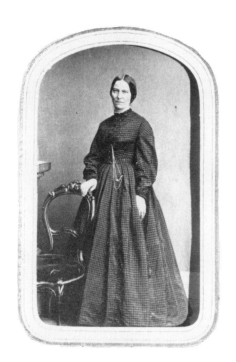

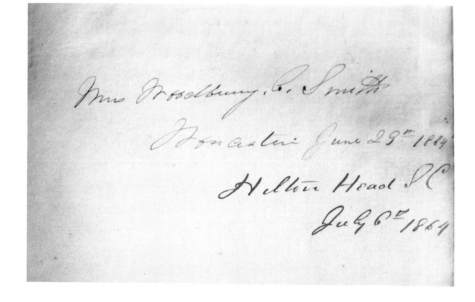

Diary kept by Nurse Smith at Hilton Head Hospital during the year 1864.

Excerpt dated Sunday, July 24, 1864, from Hilton Head Hospital.

Uniforms and Personal Equipment of the Civil War Surgeon

Since the publishing of Volume 1, many theories as to the appearance of the Civil War surgeon's uniform have been brought forth. We have no trouble with the uniform coat being of midnight blue cloth, single or double breasted, as was designated by rank. The sash was of forest green material and there is a known sword knot of the same color. Most of the Union shoulder straps were of a midnight blue field with the designation of rank present; sometimes the initials MS also were present. Recently, a shoulder strap has been shown that has a green field with the MS inside of it. As of the printing of this volume, no final word has been given regarding the authenticity of this strap. A picture is provided for your inspection. See Illustration on page 47.

On the following pages are examples of sidearms that surgeons purchased for their own protection. Since a surgeon was a non-combatant, these weapons would not have been used on the field of battle. Usually, when hospitals were overrun by the enemy, surgeons were able to continue to work on their patients. The surgeons then would be sent to a prisoner-of-war camp and wait to be exchanged.

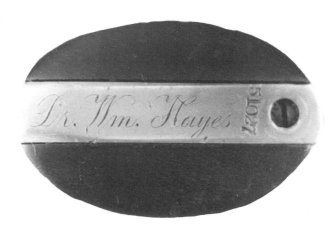

Courtesy Robert T. Lyon

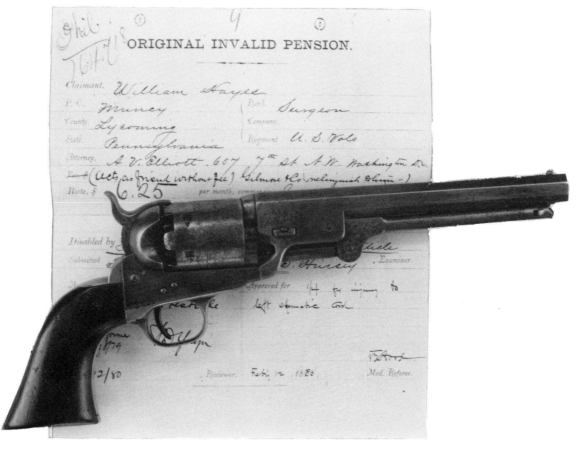

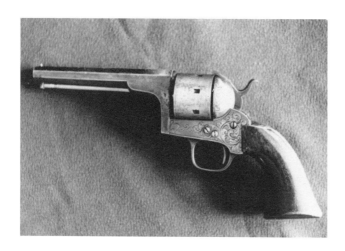

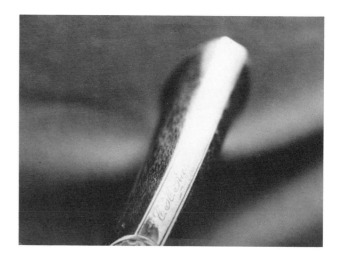

A .32-caliber Moore revolver that belonged to Surgeon Charles Richmond, who served with the 104th New York Infantry. Surgeon Richmond enlisted on August 29, 1862, and was discharged in July 1865. Surgeon Richmond was present during the Battle of Gettysburg; this weapon was in his possession.

Union surgeon's frock coat and sash, which belonged to Surgeon Fitzpatrick of the 9th Massachusetts Volunteer Infantry. Included with the coat are Fitzpatrick's medical staff sword, sword knot, leather gauntlets and a CDV of the surgeon.

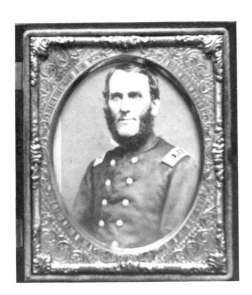

CDV of Surgeon Fitzpatrick.

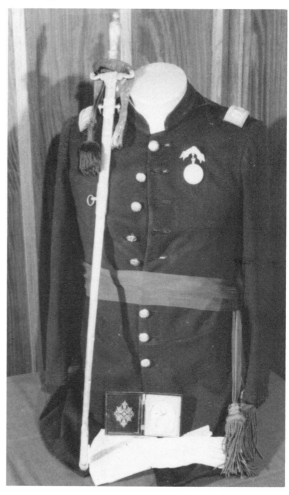

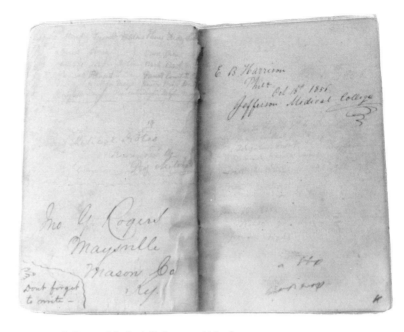

Surgeon E.B. Harrison's class schedule from Jefferson Medical College and his class notes from 1856.

Medical officer's frock coat and sword belt. This particular coat belonged to Surgeon J. Harrison of the 68th Ohio Volunteer Infantry.

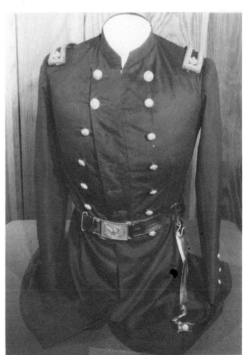

Bill of sale for uniform and accessories sold to Surgeon E.B. Harrison. The total bill was for $98.50, which included: one sword belt and sash, $50; one fatigue coat and straps, $43; one pair of gauntlets and one blanket, $5.50.

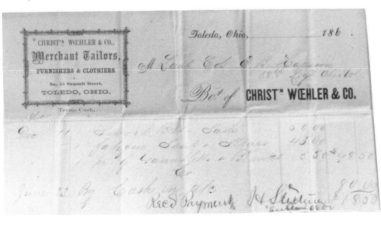

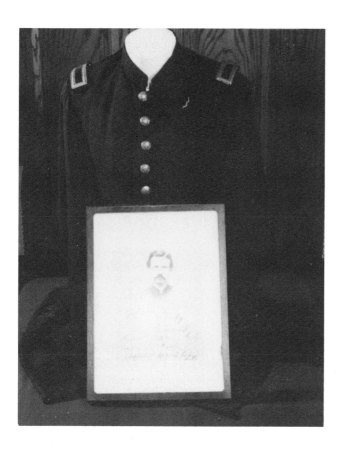

Frock coat that belonged to Surgeon Radzinsky, who
served at Hilton Head, South Carolina.

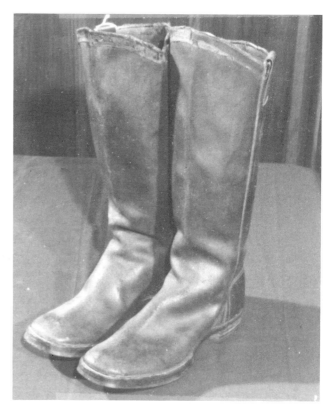

Leather boots that belonged to Surgeon Radzinsky.

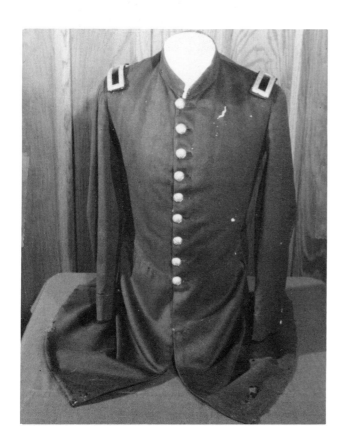

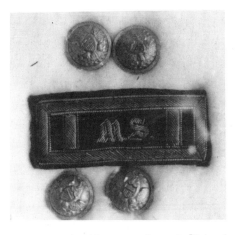

Assistant surgeon shoulder straps shown in Illustration 152 of Volume I. These straps have been identified as having belonged to Surgeon Morris of the 78th Pennsylvania Volunteer Infantry. They measure eight centimeters by three and one-half centimeters.

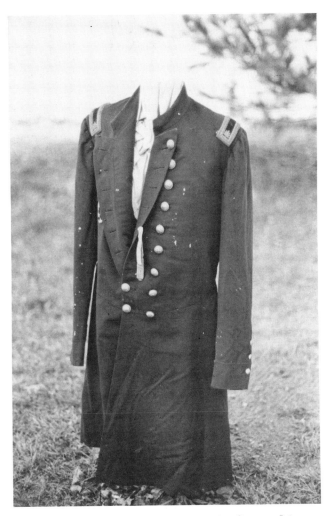

Frock coat and slouch hat that belonged to Surgeon John H. Thompson of the 124th New York Regiment. This regiment was better known as the "Orange Blossom Regiment." The ribbon attached to the lapel is orange velvet. These pictures are courtesy of Seward B. Osborne.

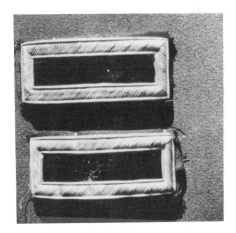

Shoulder straps of an assistant surgeon. These have a metal border.

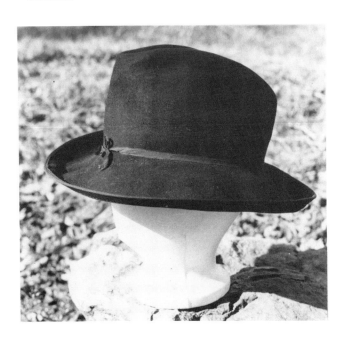

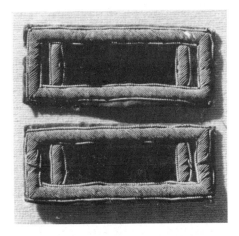

Shoulder straps of Assistant Surgeon Edgar Parker of the 13th Massachusetts Volunteer Infantry.

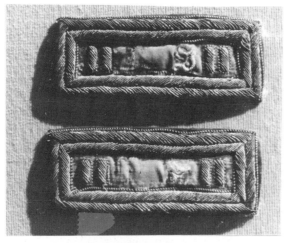

Shoulder insignia of a medical staff officer with the rank of captain. The outline of the Old English M and S can be seen. The border is gold bullion thread and the field was either blue or green.

Shoulder insignia and Hardee hat device of Surgeon Robinson of the 6th Connecticut Volunteer Infantry. These are made of very fine gold bullion thread on a midnight blue field.

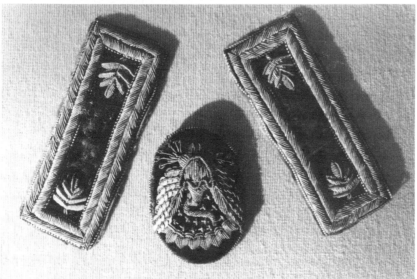

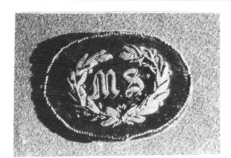

Old English MS, or Medical Staff, hat device.

Medical Staff hat device with the numerals 23 in silver bullion.

Dark green sword knot that belonged to Surgeon James Fitzpatrick of the 9th Massachusetts Infantry.

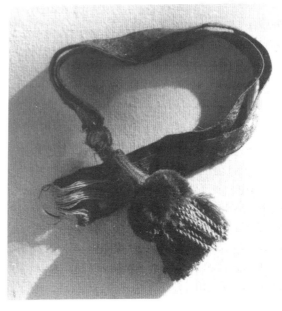

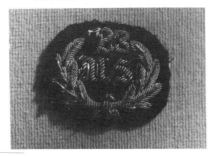

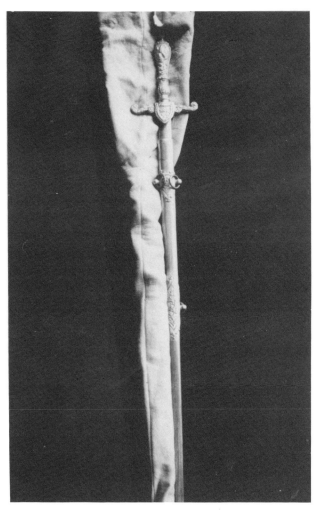

Medical officer's staff sword with original doeskin cover.

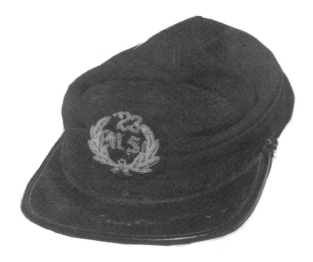

Officer's kepie with gold embroidered "MS" hat insignia. The kepie belonged to Maj. William S. Newton, O.V.I. From the collection of James Brady II.

Medical officer's slouch hat with hat cords and "U.S." embroidered insignia. The color is midnight blue.

Very fine shoulder strap with MS insignia and gold bullion border. The color of the field is green.

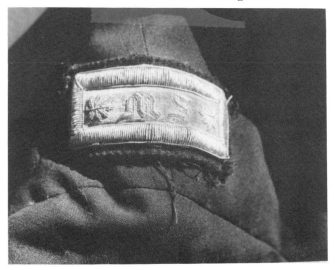

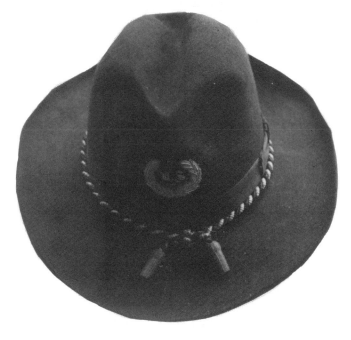

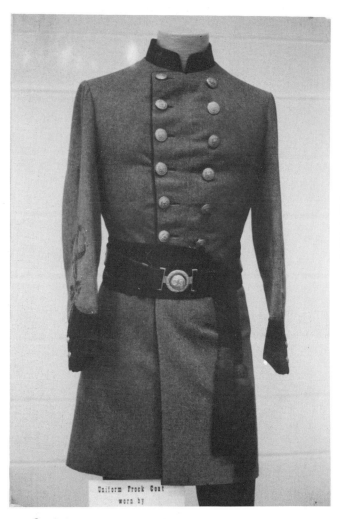

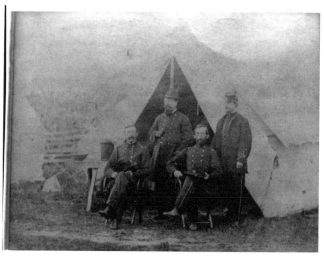

An albumin print of Surgeon John Wiley (seated at the right) in front of his tent. This was taken in 1862.

Confederate medical officer's frock coat with sash. From the collection of Dr. Thomas Wheat.

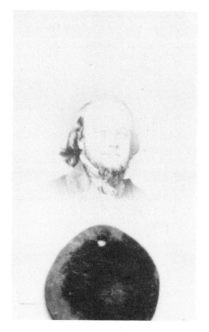

Identification disc that was worn by Surgeon Joseph A. Wolf of the 29th Pennsylvania Volunteer Infantry. This particular disc looks to be made of lead (home-made) and Wolf's initials and regiment are scratched into it. Some identification discs were made of silver and German silver. Paper tags were made by some soldiers before a battle. The CDV is of Surgeon Wolf.

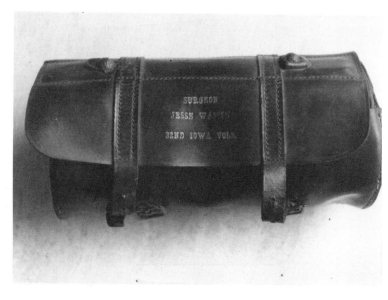

Leather valise that belonged to Surgeon Jesse Wasson of the 32nd Iowa Volunteer Infantry. It measures 10½ inches by five inches and had a handle for carrying purposes. It is round in shape and would have been used either for carrying personal belongings or bandage material. The color is brown.

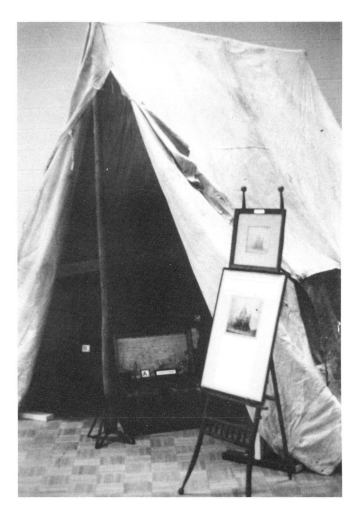

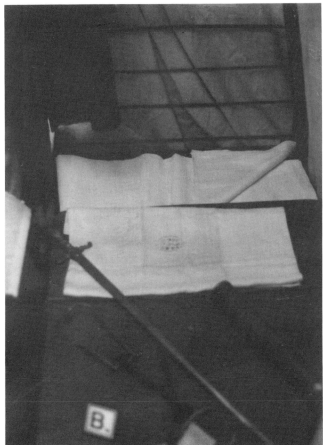

The ultimate relic of the Civil War surgeon would be his tent. The tent above belonged to Surgeon John Wiley of the 6th New Jersey Volunteer Infantry. The tent stood nine feet tall and was nine feet in length. The walls were three and one-half feet from ground to separation. It is constructed of "army duck" material and the poles were hand-fashioned. This tent was used by Surgeon Wiley from 1861 to 1864 and was present at all the major campaigns of the Army of the Potomac.

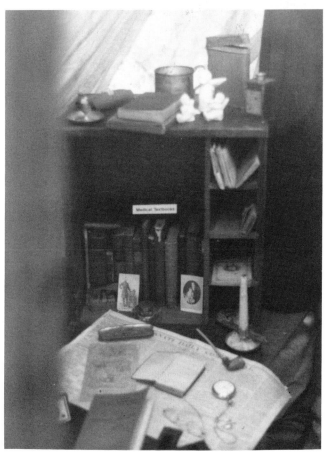

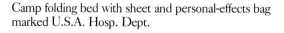
Camp folding bed with sheet and personal-effects bag marked U.S.A. Hosp. Dept.

Inside the surgeon's tent would be a camp desk and personal items.

The Hospital Steward

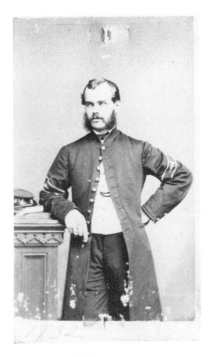

A very representative CDV showing a hospital steward wearing the regulation frock coat with appropriate insignia. This also shows what appears to be a white vest. His kepie is on the book at his right. It could be the Hospital Steward's Manual, pictured elsewhere in this chapter.

*T*he hospital steward was a non-commissioned officer. He ranked with the ordnance sergeants and was next above the first sergeant of a company. He was entitled by his rank to obedience from all enlisted men who were in hospitals, whether as patients, wardmasters, nurses or employees. In his dealings with medical officers, he never was to forget that he was an enlisted man.

His pay was $22 a month with one ration a day and the clothing allowance of an enlisted man. To be a candidate for the role of hospital steward, a man had to be between the ages of 18 and 35. He had to have competent knowledge of the English language and be able to write legibly and spell correctly. He also had to have sufficient knowledge of pharmacy to enable him to take exclusive charge of the dispensary. He also must have understood points of minor surgery regarding bandages and dressing, the extraction of teeth, and the application of cups and leeches. A knowledge of cooking enabled him to oversee the "domestic side" of hospital life.

This information came from the Hospital Steward's Manual.

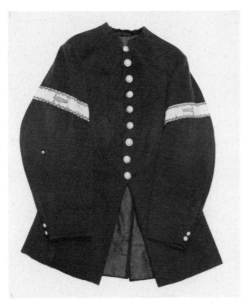

The hospital steward's coat is basically an officer's coat made from blue-black wool broad cloth. The brass buttons are those of a staff officer.

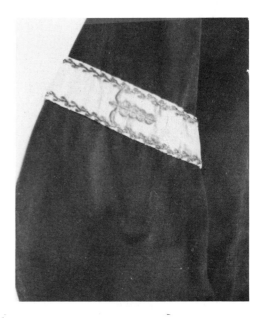

Hospital steward "half chevrons." The Army regulations of 1861 specified only that the hospital steward half chevron was to be of emerald green cloth with a yellow silk embroidered edge and caduceus. This particular coat had chevrons and caduceus of gold bullion.

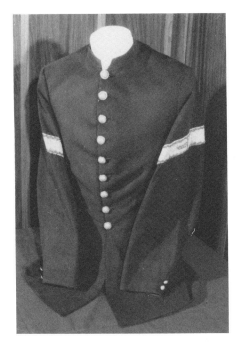

Hospital steward's frock coat, midnight blue in color with nine buttons.

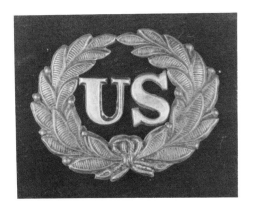

Regulation hat device of a hospital steward. On page 481 of the Revised Regulations for the Army of the United States (1861), a description of the device is given: "The wreath in front of brass, with the letters U.S. in Roman, of white metal. The hat cords will be of buff and green, mixed."

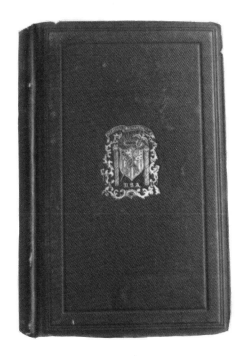

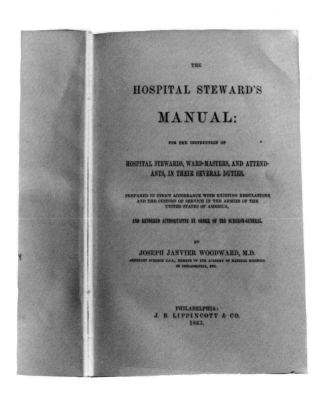

Hospital Steward's Manual written by J.J. Woodward, M.D., in 1863. On the cover is the Medical Corps insignia.

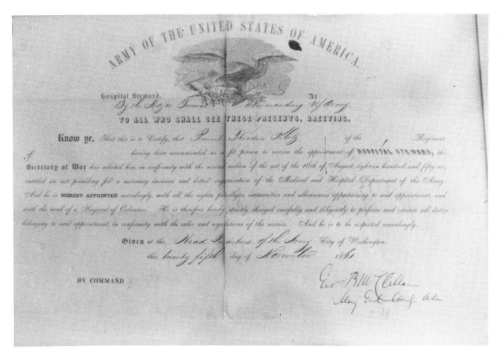

Hospital steward's commission signed by Maj. Gen. George B. McClellan. It is dated November 25, 1861.

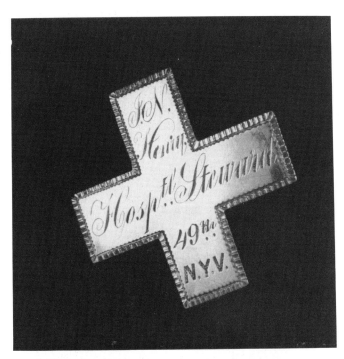

Example of a hospital steward's identification insignia. This particular insignia is made of coin silver and is one and one-quarter inches square. It belonged to Steward J.N. Henry of the 49th New York Volunteers. Courtesy of James Frasca.

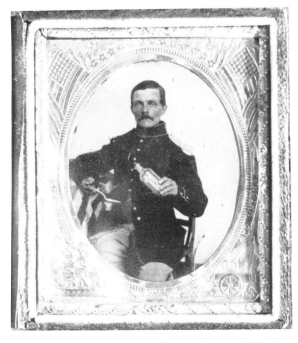

Very rare tintype of a "working" hospital steward. He is wearing a regulation frock coat with shoulder scales. He appears to be pouring material from a hospital bottle onto a spoon. The seams on the collar and cuffs would be crimson in color as per regulation.

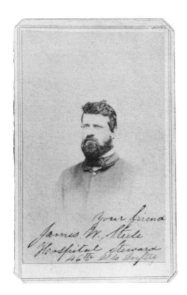

CDV of Hospital Steward James Steele of the 46th Illinois Volunteer Infantry.

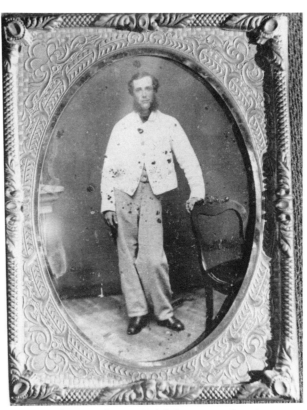

Hospital Steward Charles A. McQuesten of the 6th Maine Infantry. He is wearing a white jacket.

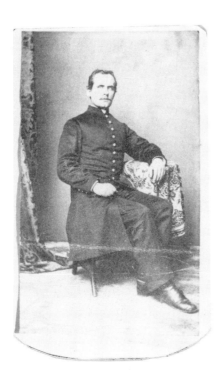

Hospital Steward Jacob Nebrich of the 2nd Division, 5th Army Corps, wearing a frock coat with no sleeve insignia.

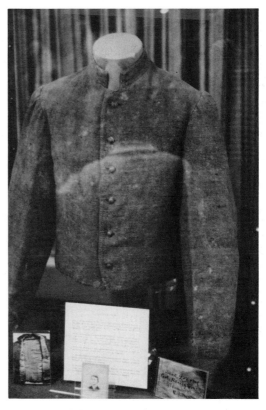

Confederate hospital steward's waist jacket of butternut cloth. Courtesy of Robt. McDonald.

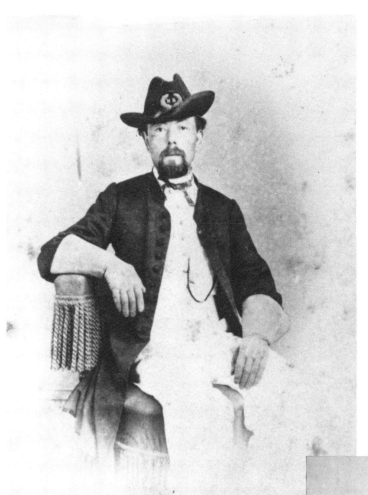

Photograph of Hospital Steward Paul Wald wearing a "regulation" chaplin's frock coat with cloth-covered buttons. He also is wearing a white vest with white trousers. Courtesy of James Frasca.

Enlarged photo of a hospital steward showing a smaller medical caduceus on what appears to be a four-button coat.

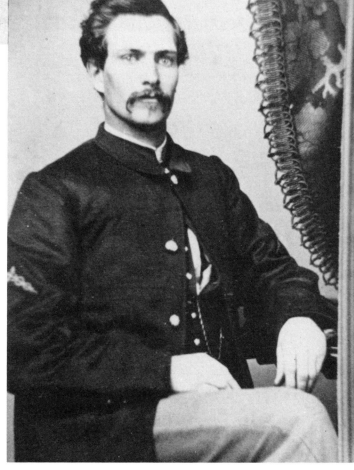

Surgical Procedure

A Pictorial Encyclopedia of Civil War Medical Instruments and Equipment dealt with the surgical techniques of the operating surgeon.

This chapter will elaborate on the problems resulting from these procedures. Sir Rickman John Godlee in 1917 wrote a volume that dealt with the life of Lord Joseph Lister. In his book, he devoted chapters to problems of healing wounds that plagued the Civil War surgeon.

Lord Lister stated that all attempts at abdominal surgery, thorax surgery and skull surgery were predestined to failure—not so much because of the techniques but because of the problems of post-operative suppuration and laudible pus. He stated: "Abdominal surgery, which after 1879 supplied a large portion of the general surgeon's work, was hardly thought of during the Civil War era."

There was only one operation performed on the thorax (chest cavity) and this was an opening of an empyema (letting out a collection of matter from the pleural, or lung cavity). The spinal canal or the cranial cavity were almost equally unexplored. Occasionally the skull was trephined or opened for the purpose of evacuating a collection of blood resulting from fractures.

Lister stated: "Any attempt to realize what teachers taught and what students learned and, in fact, what all doctors thought about hospital diseases in 1865, is as like trying to appreciate the state of mind of the inhabitants of this planet before they had begun to doubt that it was the center of the universe."[1]

In 1987, we know that disease is attributed to certain microbial agents and bacteria. In the 1860s, microbes were hardly spoken of and were not recognized as enemies but rather as "microscopic curiosities."

Erysipelas, pyaemia, septicemia and hospital gangrene were four major hospital diseases. Erysipelas, or "St. Anthony's Fire," was a common problem; few hospitals were ever totally free from it. It varied in intensity from an angry blush spreading over the face to an extensive inflammation and suppuration among the muscles—most likely fatal.

Pyaemia is the formation of clots in the veins. The clots detach and are carried by the circulation to the lungs and distant parts of the body. It often is accompanied by a "shivering fit" which is followed by others at distinctive intervals.

Septicemia was described by Civil War surgeons as "blood poisoning," which caused clotting of the venous flow of blood.

Hospital gangrene was among the great killers of the Civil War soldier. Lister, in his 1865 book, alluded to its great "awful frequency."[2] He stated that it was due to the impure state of the atmosphere produced by the overcrowding of patients with decomposing sores. Today, we understand that "hospital gangrene" is caused by a specific bacteria—streptococcus pyogenes. This disease blazed through the hospital wards and was carried by, of all things, the hands of the surgeons and wound dressings. The official records cite 2,642 cases of the "black death" of which 1,142 were fatal.[3]

In his book, Lister also mentions another disease that caused many deaths during the Civil War—tetanus. In the 1860s, this disease was almost always fatal and very painful. There was no cure because the cause was unknown until 1872, when Lister suggested that a microbe caused it. During the Civil War, it was transmitted by the surgeon's hands, surgical instruments and sponges (used to wash wounds). Because of the proximity of field hospitals to barns and livestock areas, the disease became more rampant. Lister stated: "The opportunities for the transference of disease from one patient to another were as great as the precautions to prevent it were inadequate."[4] Only after the cause was identified was the regulation of these diseases begun. During the 1860s, no theory had been brought forward that afforded a rational explanation of the nature of hospital disease. Surgeons, fighting an enemy in the dark, resigned themselves to the fact that it was inevitable.

If the Civil War had been fought in the 1870s rather than in the 1860s, probably half the fatalities could have

Footnotes

1. Godlee, Rickman John, *Lord Lister*, MacMillam and Co., London, 1917, p. 124.
2. *Ibid.*, p. 125.
3. Brooks, Stewart, *Civil War Medicine*, Charles Thomas, Springfield, 1966, p. 84.
4. Godlee, Rickman John, *Lord Lister*, MacMillam and Co., London, 1917, p. 162.

been avoided by an understanding of the work of Lister and Pasteur. On January 28, 1866, Lister wrote his father, "I am trying some more experiments with carbolic acid upon healing sores and wounds."[5]

Lister read the accounts of Pasteur, in which he stated that organisms that produce fermentation and putrefaction are carried on particles of dust floating in the atmosphere. He stated that these particles can be destroyed by *heat*, filtration and chemicals. Lister also observed that simple fractures (ones that do not cause an opening of the skin) usually healed with little or no pus formation, whereas compound fractures (those that do open the skin) almost always had a problem with pus production. This observation gave him the idea of keeping out the "floating air micro organisms" by covering the open wound with sheets of cloth and a rubber material that contained first creosote, then carbolic acid. This was the first attempt at aseptic wound dressings. On May 27, 1866, he wrote his father: "There is one of my cases in the infirmary which I am sure will interest you. It is a compound fracture of the leg with a wound of considerable size. Though hardly expecting success, I tried the application of carbolic acid to the wound so as to avoid the fearful mischief of supperation throughout the limb. Well, it is now eight days since the accident and the patient has been going on exactly as if there were no external wound, as if the fracture was a simple one."[6]

On October 20, 1866, Lister again wrote his father: "I now perform an operation for the removal of a tumour etc., with a totally different feeling from what I used to have; in fact, surgery is becoming a different thing altogether."[7]

How different surgery was to become! If only the Civil War surgeon could have been able to obtain and use this information, so much suffering and death could have been avoided.

---

5. *Ibid.*, p. 162.
6. *Ibid.*, p. 187.
7. *Ibid.*, p. 198.

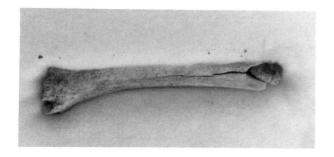

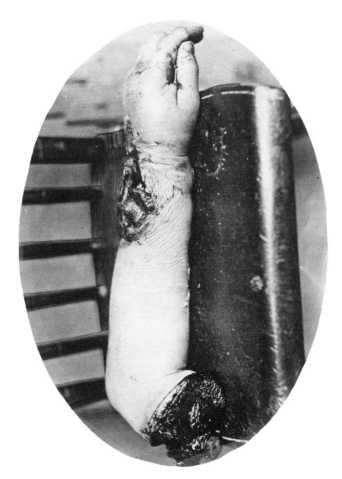

Courtesy of Armed Forces Institute of Pathology—Walter Reed Army Hospital.

Medical Instruments of the Civil War Period

*A*s gruesome as the next two illustrations are, they represent the surgical realities of the Civil War era. The illustration to the left shows the effect of a "minie ball" on the radius bone, or forearm. This conical piece of lead not only tore away flesh but when it penetrated bone, it caused a splintering effect that necessitated amputation of the limb. Before the advent of the "minie ball," the solid round ball would often bounce off the bone, causing a deep bruise or simple fracture. This was not so with the "minie ball," which, by its wedging effect, caused a multi-fractured wound that more often than not was complicated by an opening through the skin.

The ilustration above shows that the only way to treat this kind of wound was primary amputation. We see by this photo a telescoping surgical technique whereby the bone is severed high above the incision line, thereby causing a stump that had a great deal of soft tissue around it. This made for a comfortable stump when wearing the necessary prosthesis.

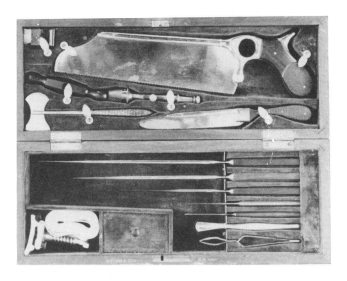

Large surgical kit marked Shepard and Dudley, New York. Courtesy of Alex Peck.

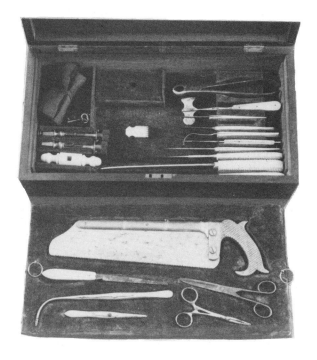

Early surgical kit (1830-1840) that is marked Goulding, N.Y. Notice the ivory-handled instruments and the brass handle of the amputation saw. Courtesy of Alex Peck.

Very large and complete amputation kit marked Tiemann. The lid of the case is marked USA Hosp. Dept. Courtesy of Alex Peck.

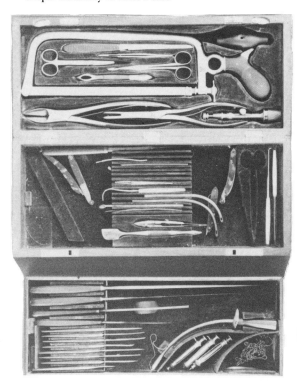

Capital amputation kit (made by Stoddard), which belonged to Surgeon Harrison of the 68th Ohio Volunteer Infantry.

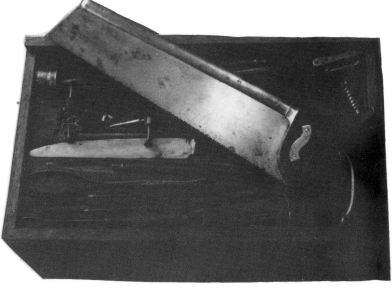

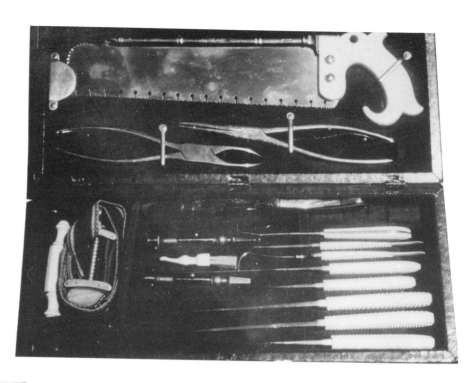

Very fine and ornate surgical kit of the 1850-1860s. This kit was made by Goulding and has ivory handles. This type of kit was probably not military but shows the type of workmanship that went into a fine piece of medical equipment. Courtesy of Alex Peck.

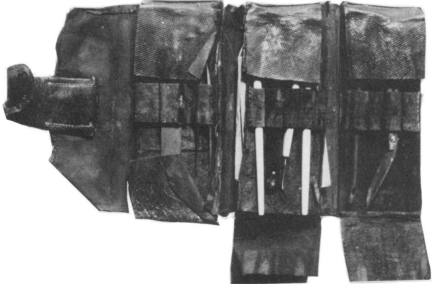

Examples of folding or "pocket" surgical kits used by surgeons during the Civil War.

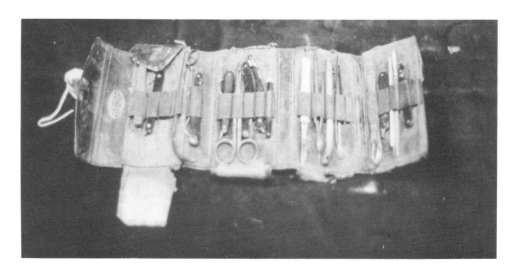

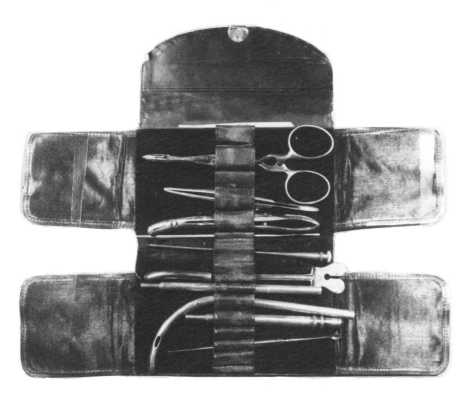

Pocket surgical kit.

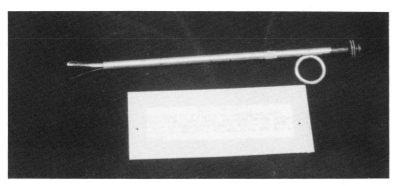

Two examples of bullet or foreign body forceps used by the Civil War surgeon. The illustration above is unique because the "fingers" come out of the barrel to engage the bullet.

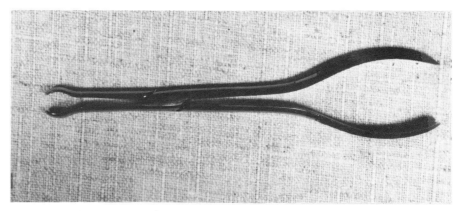

Courtesy of Rev. Norman Bowen.

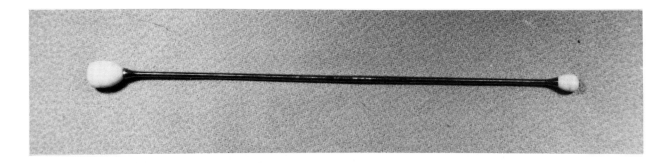

Two types of the Nelanton probe. The porcelain tips make it easier to detect a metal object which would leave gray marks on the white porcelain. Courtesy of Rev. Bowen.

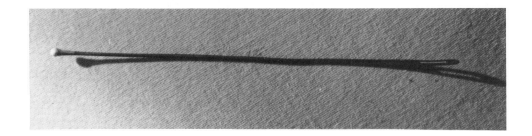

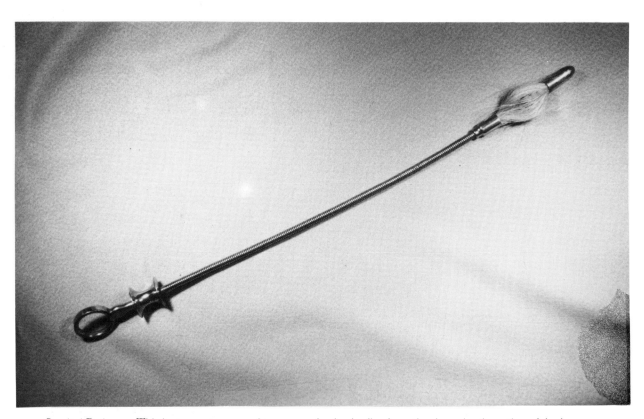

Surgical Probang—This instrument was used to remove foreign bodies from the throat by the action of the horse-hair bristles on the end. Courtesy of Rev. Bowen.

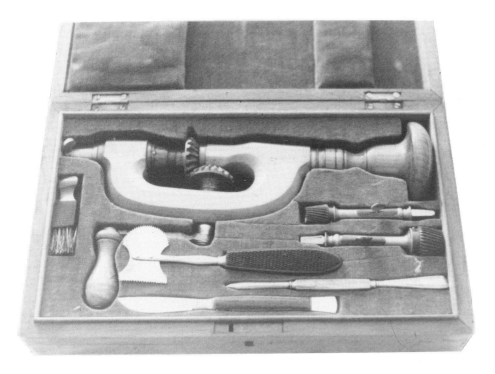

Trepanning kit used for cranial surgery. Unlike the trephine that was turned by a twisting motion, this instrument used the action of a drill. Inside the kit is also a Hey's saw, scalpel, periosteal elevator and brush.

Examples of hard rubber syringes. The upper syringe was used to treat gonorrhea by injecting substances such as silver nitrate into the penis. The lower syringe, with a brass needle attached, most likely was used to inject pain-killing substances under the skin. Usually, morphine was mixed with water and injected by this type of syringe.

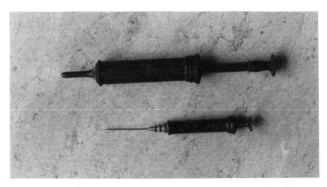

Early type of rectal or axillary thermometer.

Solid ivory-handled knife used for vaccination.

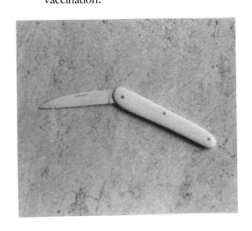

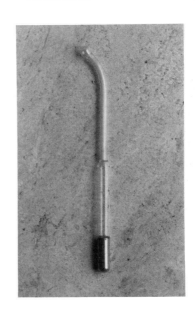

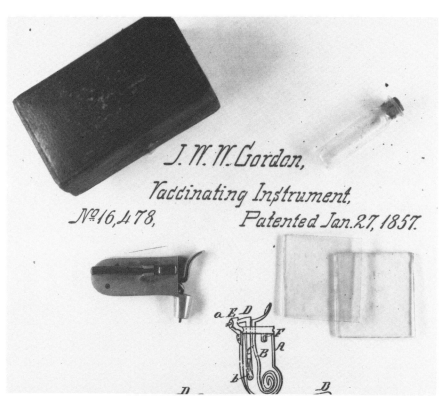

Civil War era vaccinating instrument, patented in 1857. From the collection of Dr. Terry Hambrecht.

Copy of the original patent diagram for the Lambert Tourniquet, dated 1862. This was the belt-buckle type of tourniquet.

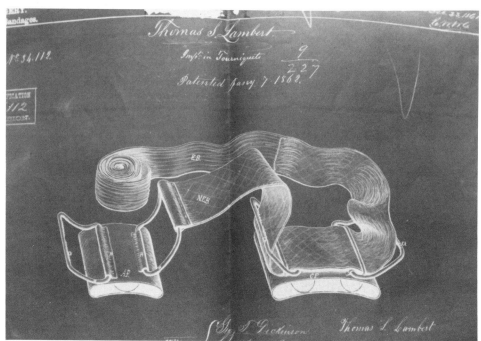

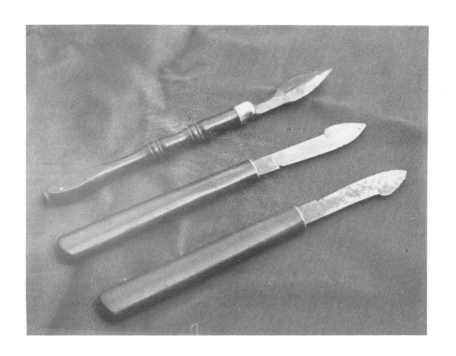

Since the publishing of Volume I of the *Pictorial Encyclopedia of Civil War Medical Instruments and Equipment*, much controversy has arisen over the photo of the pocket kit (Illustration 40) and the photo of the venesection knives (Illustration 63). They are reproduced again in this volume.

It has been pointed out that there were devices with the same configuration as the knives that were shown; however, they were used as ink erasers. Conversely, many devices that looked like ink erasers were used as scalpels or venesection devices. Consider the roll-up kit as proof. This kit had the instruments in place and the outline of each instrument pressed into the leather holder. They were not substituted at a later date.

Next, consider the medical notes of Surgeon Harrison of the 68th Ohio. He attended Jefferson Medical College in 1856-57. His class notes from Dr. Pancoast's lecture show a drawing of a "scalpel." The notes state that fine scalpels can be fashioned from inexpensive "document changers."

Scalpels or ink erasers?
The three pictured together probably are ink erasers. The one in the surgical kit was used as a scalpel, and those pictured in Smith's Surgical text of 1858 show different variations.

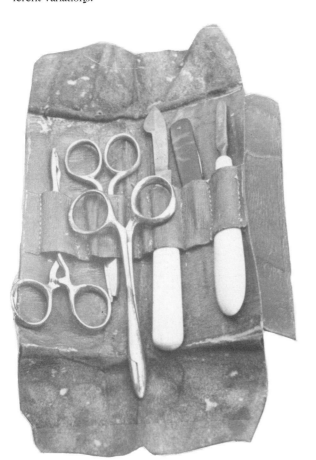

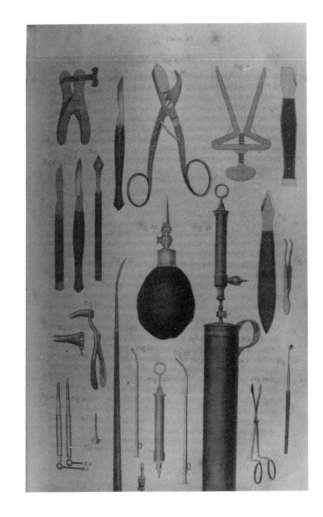

Medical Equipment Used During the Civil War

*T*he medical kit illustrated here is the U.S. Army Medicine Pannier that was put together by Squibb and sold to the Army for $110. The following items are contained in this kit:

 1. Cantharides
 2. Silver nitrate
 3. Silver chloride
 4. Iodine
 5. Tartar emetic
 6. Mercurous chloride
 7. Beef extract
 8. Coffee extract
 9. Condensed milk
10. Black tea
11. Alcohol
12. Spirit of ether
13. Strong alcohol
14. Cough mixture
15. White sugar
16. Chloroform
17. Liniment
18. Syrup of squill
19. Ammonia water
20. Compound spirit of ether
21. Tincture of opium
22. Fluid extract of cinchona
23. Fluid extract of valerian
24. Fluid extract of ginger
25. Olive oil
26. Oil of turpentine
27. Glycerine
28. Paregoric
29. Solution of ferric sulfate
30. Spirit of ammonia
31. Compound cathartic pills
32. Pills of colocynth and ipecac
33. Ipecac and opium powder
34. Quinine sulfate
35. Potassium chlorate
36. Potassium bicarbonate
37. Potassium iodide
38. Rochelle salt
39. Morphine sulfate
40. Pills of camphor and opium
41. Mercury pills
42. Opium pills
43. Tannic acid
44. Alum
45. Collodion
46. Creosote
47. Fluid extract of aconite
48. Fluid extract of colchicine
49. Fluid extract of ipecac
50. Tinc. of ferric chloride
51. Lead acetate
52. Zinc sulfate

U.S. Army Medicine Pannier that was manufactured by Edward R. Squibb, M.D.

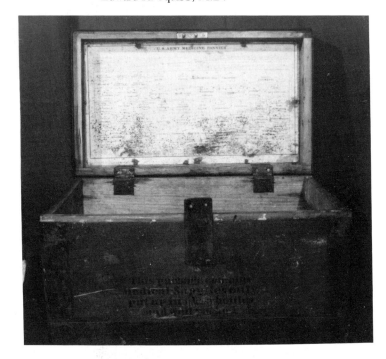

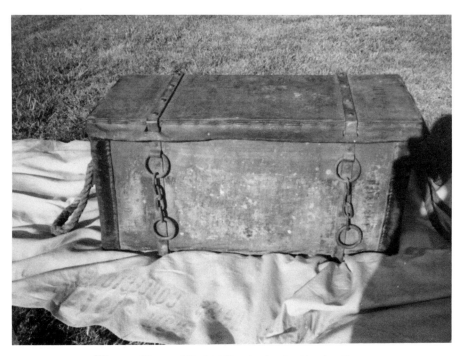

The rare Dunton Medical Pannier for the Cavalry. From the collection of Frank Bennett.

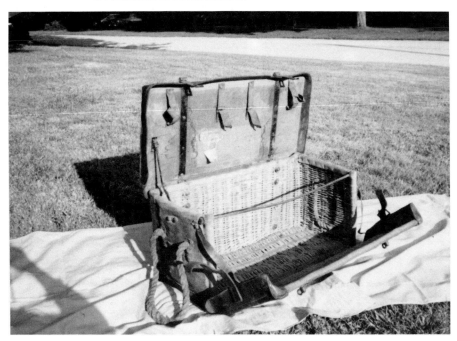

Early 1858 period medical panniers were wooden and covered with tarred linen. Later, around 1860, they were modified by McEvoy's patent No. 34117. They were of wicker with top and frontal openings, and they were covered with painted canvas cloth. This combination was both lighter and stronger.

Jacob Dunton Jr. was a pharmacist on Market Street in Philadelphia in the 1820s. He had several patents for special tourniquets, medicine bottles, pack saddles, a medical wagon and other medical supplies. Following in his father's footsteps, Dunton began working with Surgeon General Hammond equipping the medical supplies in the knapsack and panniers of the Army regiments. The price per pannier was $100.00 for the container and $250 for its contents. The weight of the pannier and its contents was 80 pounds.

In 1863, Dunton fell out of favor with the surgeon general's office. Edward R. Squibb, M.D., was named as medical supplier. Courtesy of Frank Bennett.

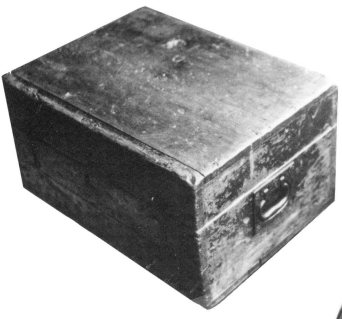

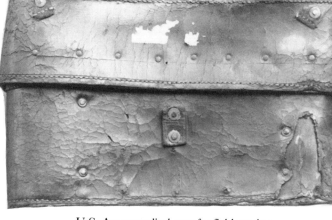

U.S. Army medical case for field service.
31 cm × 17 cm × 15 cm. Black leather.

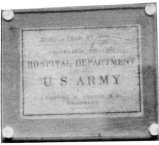

Wooden medicine box that was manufactured by Edward R. Squibb, M.D. This box probably contained chemicals for anesthesia—chloroform or ether.

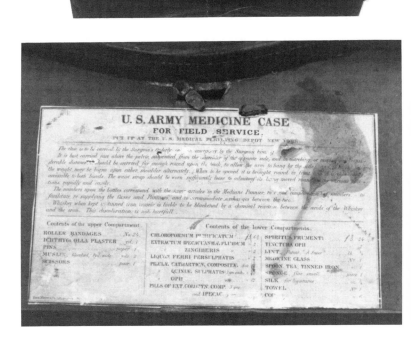

Close-up of table of contents of field medical case.

24 roller bandages
1 yd. ichthyocolla plaster
1 Paper of Pins
2 yds. bleached muslin
1 pair scissors

Chloroform
Ipecac extract
Zinc sulphate
Ferric sulphate
Quinine sulphate
Opii
Pills of Colocyn Comp.—3 grs.
Pills of Ipecac—1/2 grs.

UPPER COMPARTMENT

Used primarily for wound bandaging

Spiritus Frumenti
Opii tincture
Lint
Medicine glass
Teaspoon Tinned Iron
Sponge
Silk (suture)
Towel

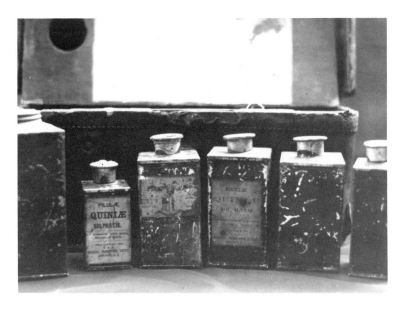

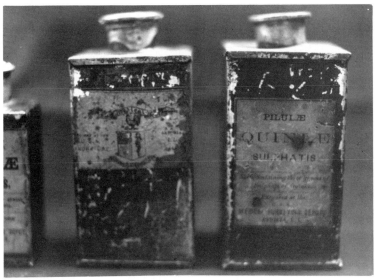

Some of the tinned medicine containers found in the field medical case. Tin marked quinine sulphate is 10.5 cm ×5 cm ×5 cm. The smaller tin marked quinine is 8.5 cm ×3.5 cm × 3.5 cm. All have cork stoppers except the large one on the left (top picture). It has a screw top and measures 12.5 cm ×6 cm ×6 cm.

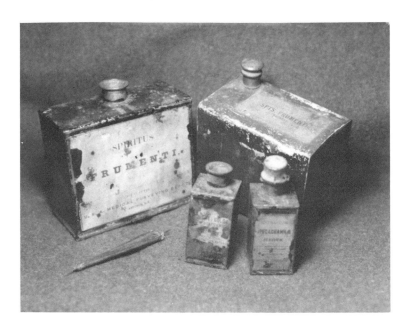

Medicine containers found in the U.S. Army medicine case for field service. The two larger tins contain spirits frumenti or fermenti (hospital whiskey or alcohol). The tin on the lower right contains extract of ipecac. Courtesy of Dr. Thomas Sweeney.

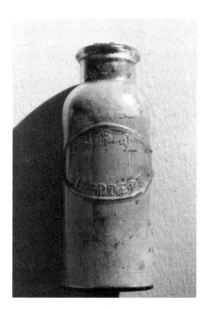
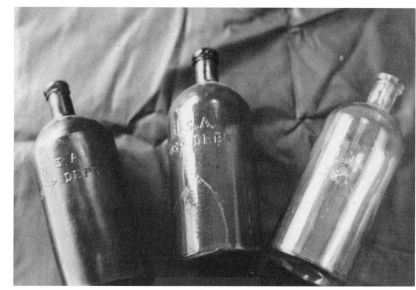

Amber and green medical bottles of the Civil War era. All are marked U.S.A. Hosp. Dept.

Anatomical teaching device that shows some of the bones of the hand, wrist, and one bone of the fore-arm. On the back of the wooden holder is the mark-ing U.S. Hosp. Dept.—1863. This was probably used to teach hospital stewards, nurses, and perhaps even surgeons about the anatomy of the forearm, hand and wrist.

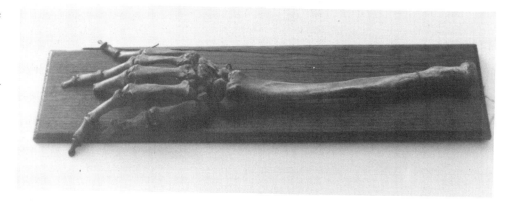

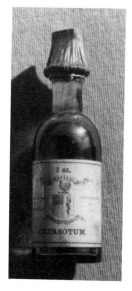

Bottle marked Creasotum. It has the original contents and the "onion skin" seal. Creosote was used as a remedy against hospital gangrene.

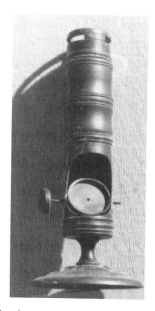

A microscope made of hard rubber and used during the Civil War era.

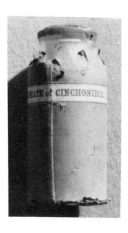

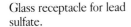

Glass bottle for cinchona, which had "aspirin-like" qualities. It was given to combat fevers.

Glass receptacle for lead sulfate.

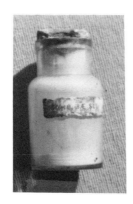

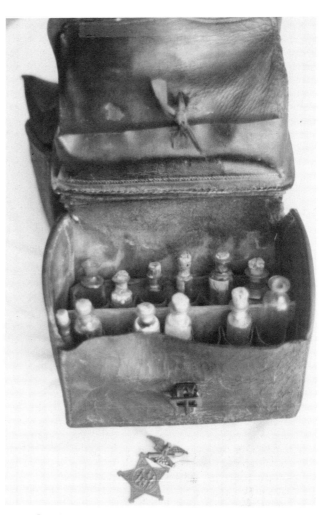

Leather saddle bags with original bottles of medicine. Included with the saddle bags was a GAR medal. Unfortunately, the saddle bags were not identified.

Small medical canteen. This canteen is 4½ inches in diameter and ¾-inch wide. It is a very crudely made item with three loops for a strap.

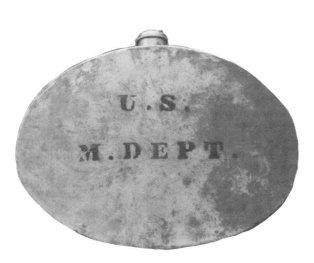

Oval or "kidney bean" medical canteen. Marked U.S. Med. Dept., the canteen is 24 cm × 16.5 cm, and has a brass screw stopper.

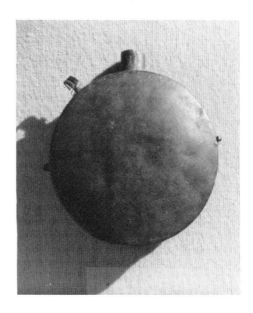

Common canteen that was used by a surgeon for quinine preparations.

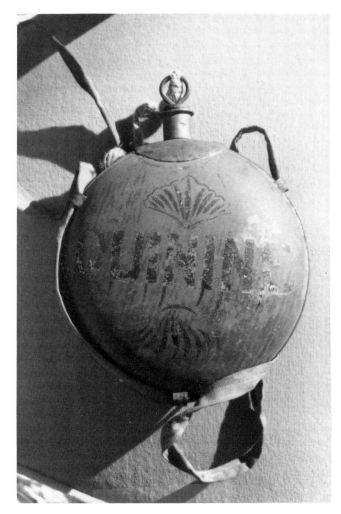

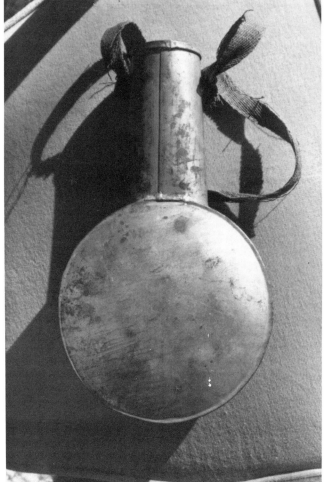

Canteen that has been described as a medical canteen. This is questionable. It has a very wide mouth, 2¼ inches in diameter, and a period strap. Collectors still are looking for a definite identification of this canteen.

Ambulance Corps

*E*stablishment of a uniform ambulance corps system in the armies of the United States was not accomplished until the spring of 1864, when, by an act of Congress, the authority of the Medical Department over the Ambulance Corps was fully established. How effectively the medical officers used the power thus conferred is well shown in the systematic manner in which the immense number of wounded were cared for on the battlefield, removed to field or base hospitals, and distributed to general hospitals throughout all parts of the North after the battles of Wilderness, Spotsylvania Court House, Cold Harbor, Petersburg and the Georgia Campaign. The country owes a great debt to Surgeon Letterman and Surgeon Generals Hammond and Barnes for their efforts in this work.

These numbers speak for themselves: After Gettysburg, 20,342 came under the care of medical officers in a matter of days. After Wilderness and Spotsylvania, 41,000 were cared for and distributed in a matter of days.

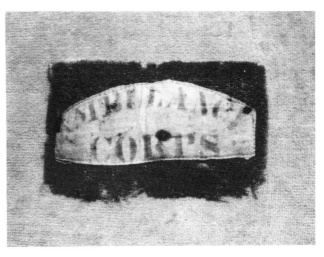

Distinctive armband used by members of the Ambulance Corps.

One of the few four-wheeled ambulances still in existence. Can be seen at Abraham Lincoln University Museum at Harrogate, Tenn.

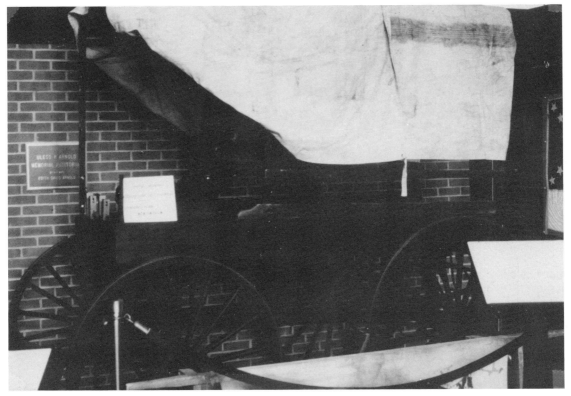

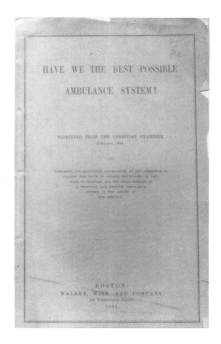

Booklet printed in 1864 by the U.S. Christian Commission that delves into the workings of the Union Ambulance System.

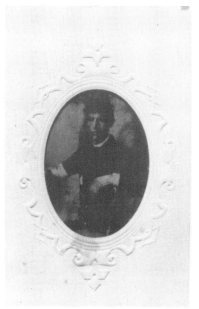

A very rare tintype of what appears to be a member of the Ambulance Corps. He is wearing a distinctive armband on his right arm. He also looks as if he is wearing white gloves.

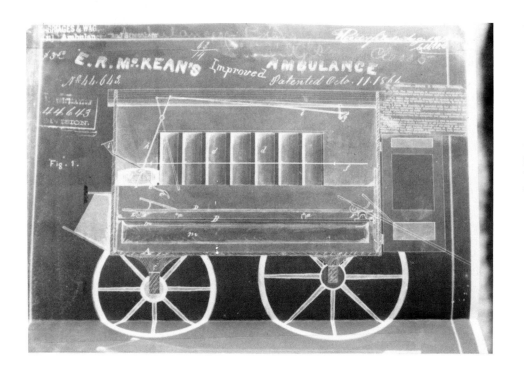

Copy of the original patent for the McKean's four-wheeled ambulance. It was dated October 11, 1864.

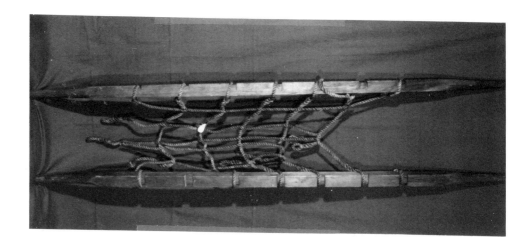

Rope stretcher used during the Civil War.

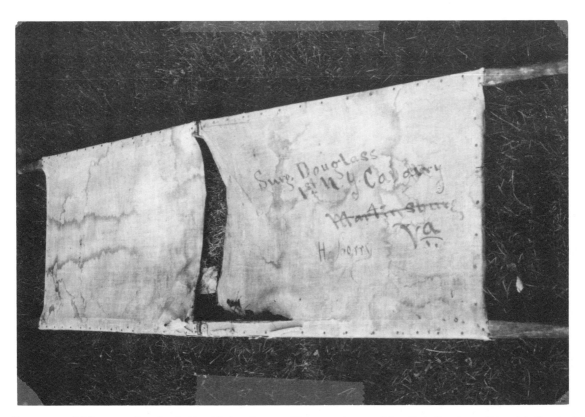

Canvas-type folding stretcher that is identified to Surgeon Douglas of the 1st New York Cavalry or "Lincoln's Cavalry."

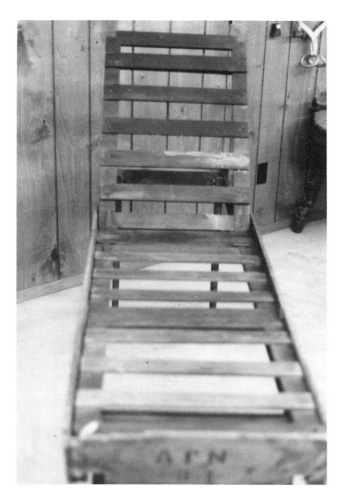 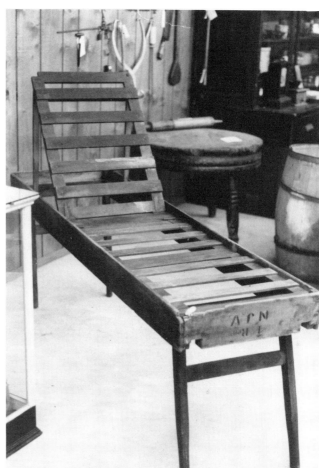

Wooden Satterlee-type stretcher. This is a unique device because it can be used as a stretcher and also as a hospital bed.

A pressed type of wood splint that was used to fixate the wrist area. The fingers would grasp the handle and the splint would form around the forearm.

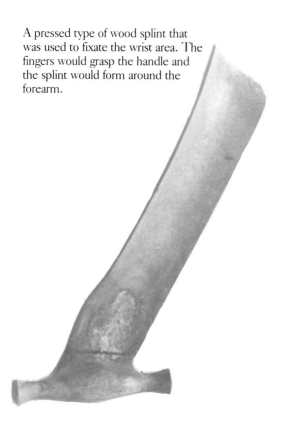

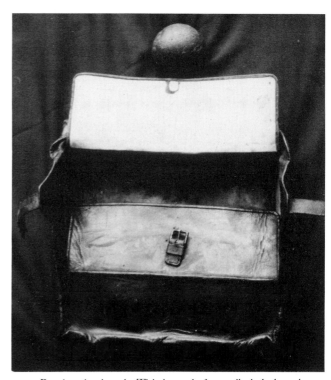

Bandage backpack: This is made from oiled cloth and was used by ambulance or stretcher personnel to carry bandage material.

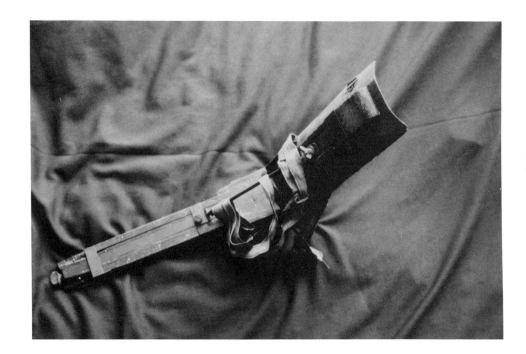

Splints that were used to stabilize the arm after resection surgery. They have hinges and the degree of healing angle can be varied.

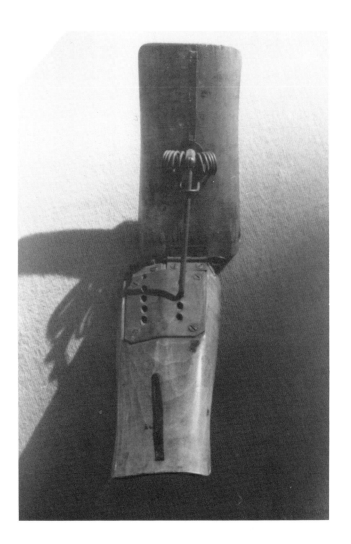

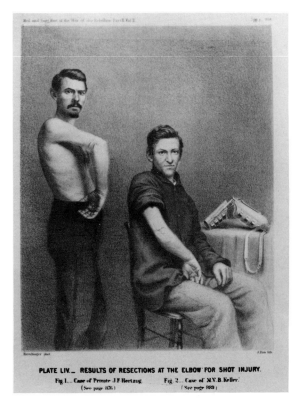

PLATE LIV.— RESULTS OF RESECTIONS AT THE ELBOW FOR SHOT INJURY.
Fig 1.— Case of Private J F Hertzog.   Fig 2.— Case of M.V.B. Keller.
(See page 876.)   (See page 889.)

Lithograph showing the hinged splint and the healed wound.

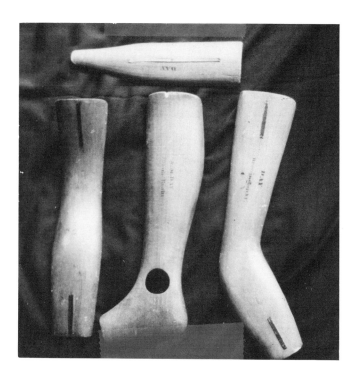

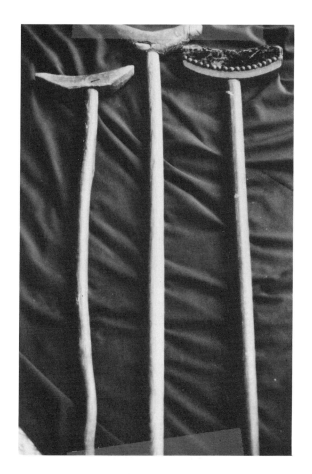

Three different types of crutches used by wounded soldiers. The one on the left is all wood, the middle one has a padded leather crotch, and the right one has a carpet-like material padding the crotch.

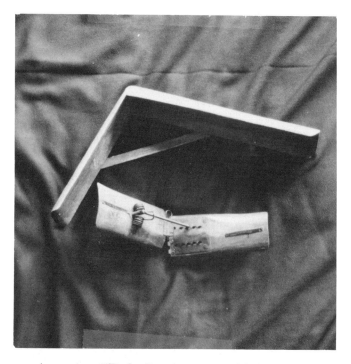

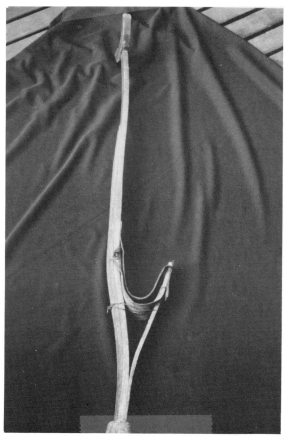

A grouping of "Day" splints that were used during the Civil War. Day was from Vermont, and he acquired patent rights to these splints.

A crutch and artificial leg combination. The stump of the lower leg fit into the crotch area.

Dental Instruments Used During the Civil War

*T*he dental profession was in its infancy during the Civil War era. New though it was, dental treatment was needed by the Civil War soldier. In the Union Army, 5,230 recruits of the 255,188 who were examined were excused from service because of poor teeth.

Surgeon General William A. Hammond stated: "No one can be healthy whose teeth are deficient or in bad condition; soldiers require that these organs should be sound. The loss of the front teeth prevents the soldier from tearing his cartridge and the loss or carious state of the molars seriously interferes with the proper mastication of his food."

How was the soldier to keep his teeth in good health? There was no organized dental corps in either Army at this time. Surgeons would try to extract offending teeth or lance gum boils. When the Army would set up a fixed camp, civilian dentists would set up clinics to care for the dental needs of soldiers. Dr. W. Leigh Burton, a dentist who treated the troops, outlined his day: "In addition to treatment of fractures of the face, the day's work consisted of from 20 to 30 fillings, the extraction of 15 to 20 teeth and the removal of tartar."

The illustrations on the following pages represent the instruments used for extraction and for filling and cleaning of Civil War soldiers' teeth.

Posed tintype of a Civil War era dentist extracting a tooth from a not-so-cooperative patient. In the closeup, notice the supply of extraction forceps and elevators in the case on the table.

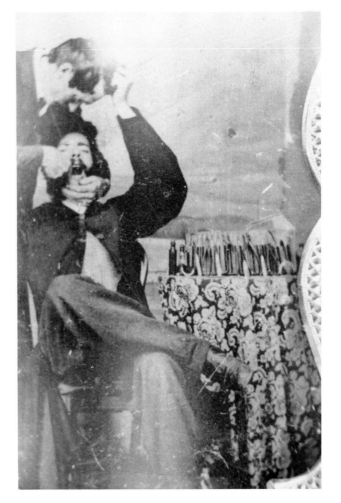

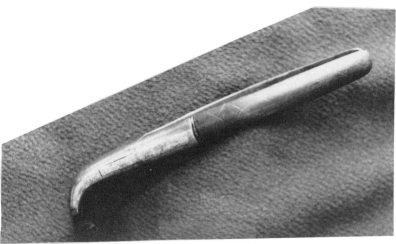

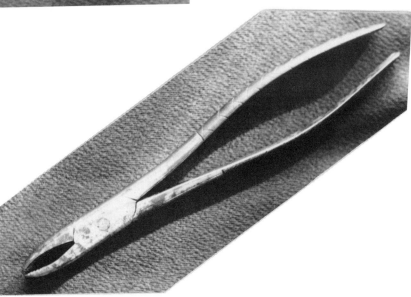

Instruments used for extraction during the 1860s. The above illustrations are forceps. The bottom illustration is an example of the extraction key. The use of the key in extraction ended with the advent of forceps.

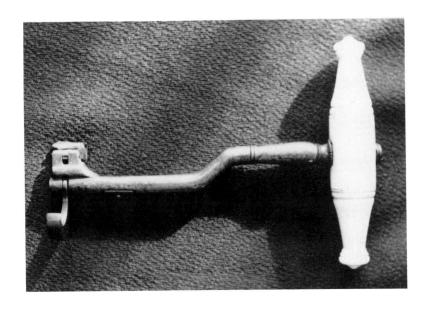

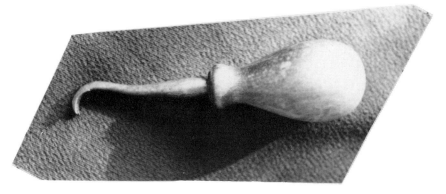

Examples of extraction elevators used during the Civil War era. These particular elevators have wooden handles. An elevator is used to wedge or pry teeth or roots out rather than to grasp and pull.

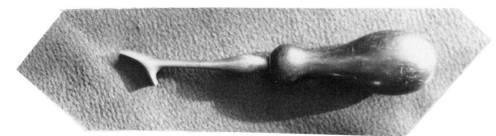

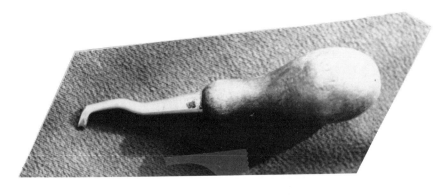

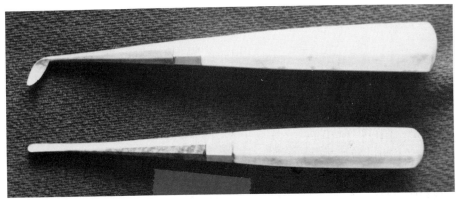

More examples of extraction elevators. The top four have ivory handles while the bottom two have ebony handles.

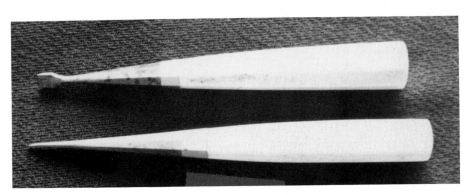

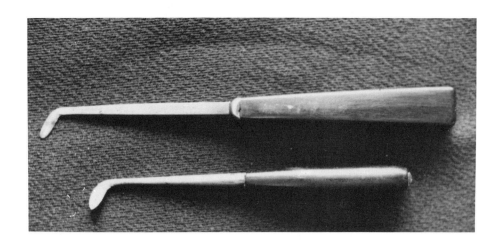

When roots of teeth had to be extracted, which happened many times after the extraction key was used, these "screw elevators" were employed. These would be screwed into the center of the root and the root was lifted out—hopefully!

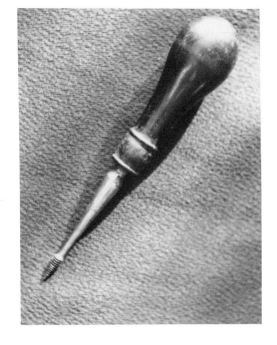

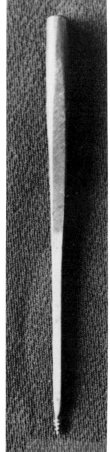

This is an example of an oral hygiene kit used in the early 19th century. The different scalers (scrapers) would be inserted into the ivory handle and deposits on the teeth and root surface would be removed by a push-pull motion. Today, these deposits are known as plaque and calculus.

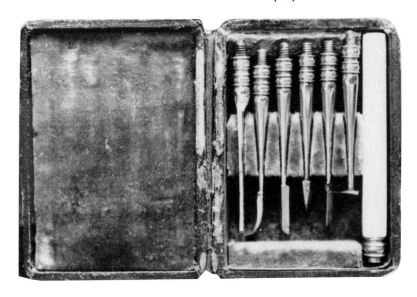

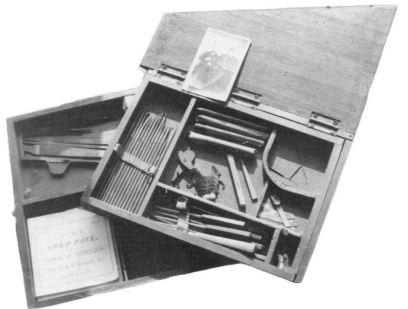

The Portable Dental Restorative Kit pictured was used to restore teeth rather than extract them. Teeth that had cavities were restored with either tin or gold foil. After the soft caries had been cleaned out of the tooth and suitable undercuts had been made, the tin or gold foil was pressed piece by piece into the preparation. When the defect was fully "plugged," the metal was smoothed or burnished.

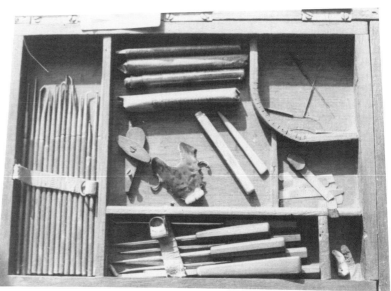

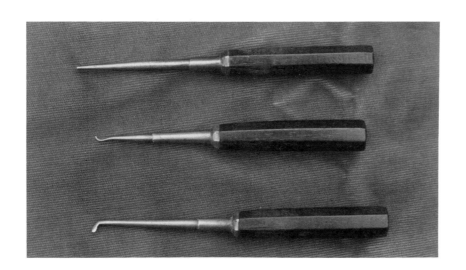

Excavators and pluggers used to restore teeth.

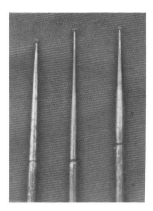

"Finger drills" that were used to open the cavity to a larger shape so it could be filled.

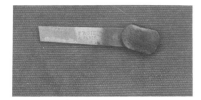

Small file used to smooth the restorations after they were placed.

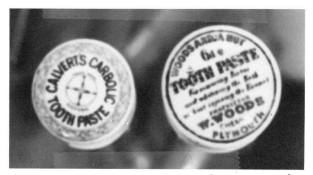

Ivory vials containing toothpaste or tooth powder. The formula for a tooth powder as described in the 1864 Treatise on Pharmacy was: powdered chalk, powdered myrrh, orris root and red chalk.

Partial denture that replaced the upper two front teeth. It is constructed of German silver and ivory teeth.

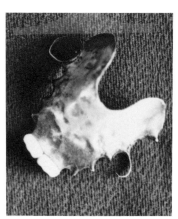

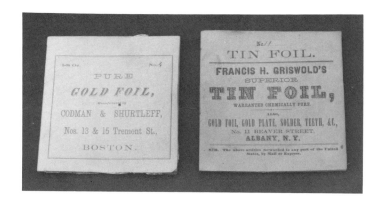

Sheets of gold or tin foil that were used to restore carious teeth.

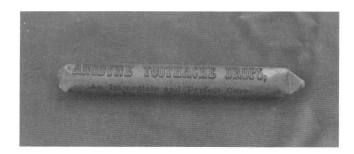

Anodyne "toothache drops" were commonly known as oil of cloves. Placed inside a carious lesion, they gave some pain control.

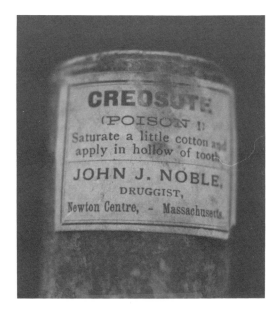

An attempt to preserve teeth was made with use of primitive root-canal therapy or endodontics. Creosote "mummified" the pulp tissue, thereby "saving" the tooth.

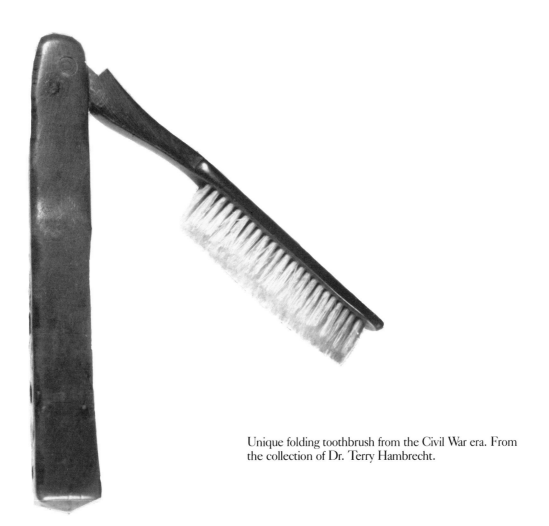

Unique folding toothbrush from the Civil War era. From the collection of Dr. Terry Hambrecht.

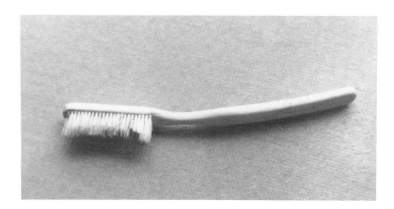

Toothbrush made of ivory handle and pig-hair bristles that was commonly used by soldiers during the Civil War.

Embalming

It is because of the Civil War that the profession of mortuary science became prevalent. The requests of families to have the bodies of their loved ones transported home for proper memorial services made it necessary for a system of preservation to become a new profession.

The Physician's Pocket Memorandum published in 1869 by C.H. Cleveland, M.D., describes the way bodies were preserved in the 1860s: "A strong solution of the chloride of zinc—1/2 ounce of the salt to a quart of alcohol and water—may be employed directly into the artery to prevent decomposition. Creosote is sometimes used as an anti-putrefactive agent, but its odor is objectionable. . . . With a common pewter syringe, it may be thrown into the arterial system, the nozzle of the instrument being introduced into a slit made in the femoral artery.

"It is customary to transport bodies in metallic burial cases, or heavy wooden boxes lined with zinc plates."

Before the War there was no need for this type of service. Public pressure demanded the ascendancy of the profession of mortuary science.

In Volume I, the embalming pump was misrepresented by what we now know as an enema pump. An embalming apparatus used during the 1860s still is being sought.

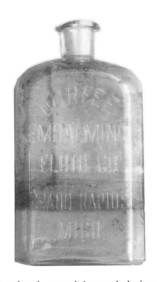

Glass bottle containing embalming fluid

Marked: Durfee
    Embalming Fluid Co.
    Grand Rapids
    Mich.

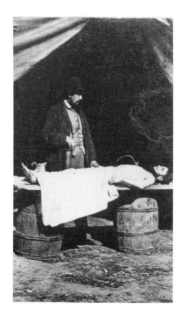

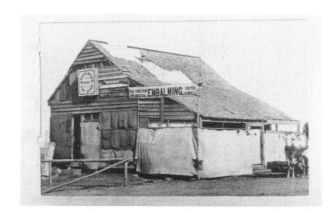

Two CDVs offering classic views of the Civil War-era embalmer and his work place.

Medical Documents of the Civil War

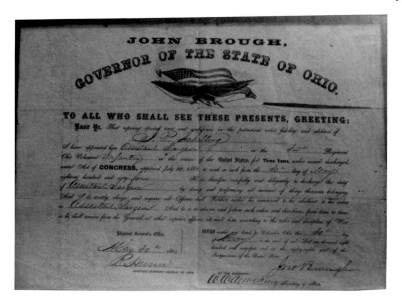

Surgeon's commission signed by the governor of Ohio, John Brough.

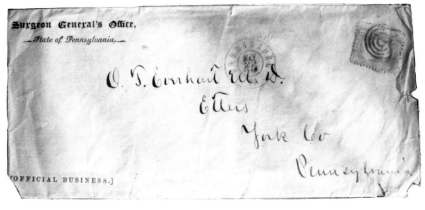

Document dated January 29, 1863, appointing Dr. O.T. Everhart assistant surgeon of a Pennsylvania regiment. It was signed by J. King, surgeon general of Pennsylvania. The accompanying envelope is also pictured.

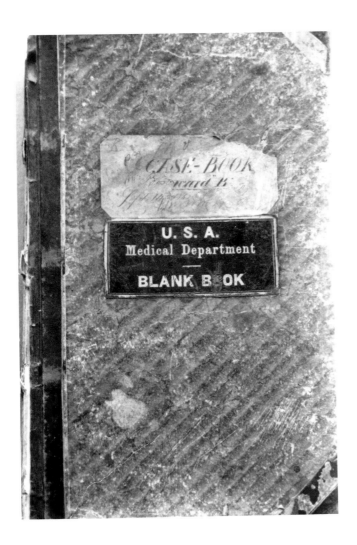

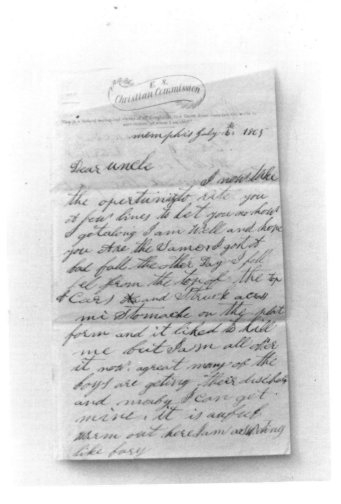

Soldier's letter written on U.S. Christian Commission stationery.

Hospital "day book" from Philadelphia Hospital, which was located on Broad and Cherry Street. The account of the wounded is from the Battle of Gettysburg.

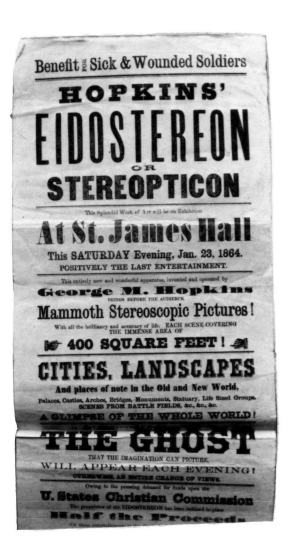

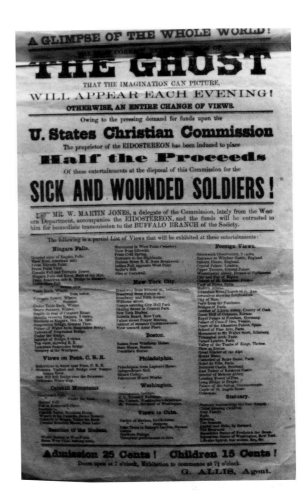

A broadside advertising an entertainment that would benefit the U.S. Christian Commission. The funds derived from these shows went to purchase items for soldiers.

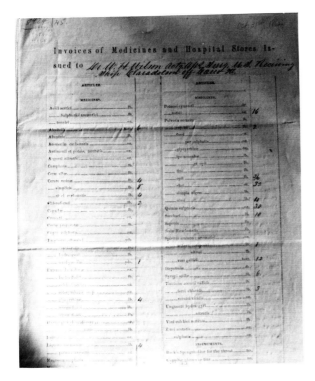

Invoice of medical and hospital stores.

One of many reports written by the U.S. Sanitary Commission on different aspects of the medical care of soldiers.

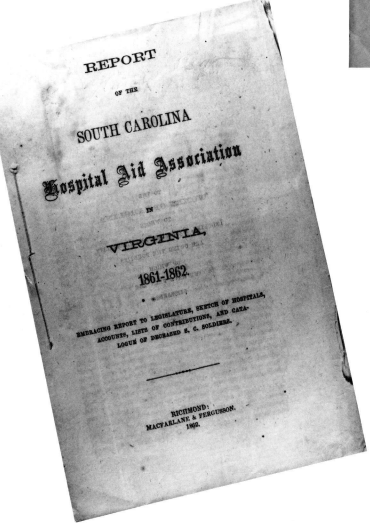

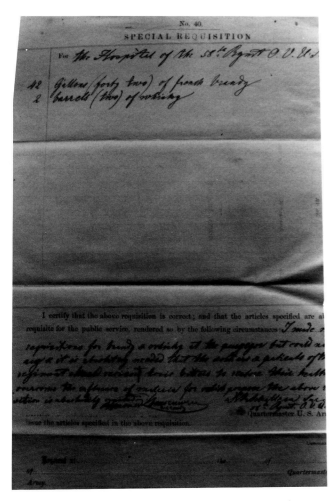

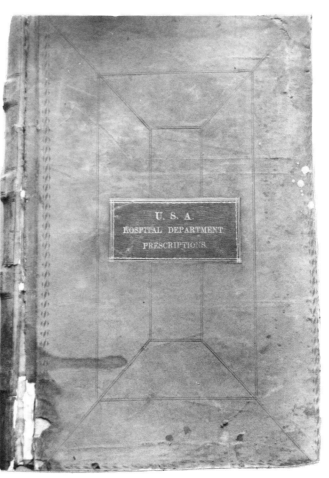

Large leather book that has a red label affixed—"U.S.A. Hospital Department Prescriptions."

Very interesting requisition for 42 gallons and 2 barrels of French brandy and whiskey for medical purposes. This was signed by the surgeon of the 58th Ohio Volunteer Infantry.

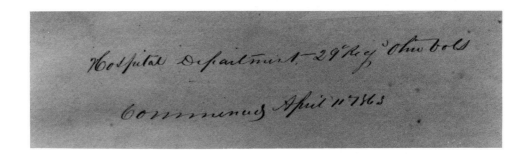

Inscription from the book that contained the prescription records of the 29th Ohio Volunteer Infantry. It is dated April 1863.

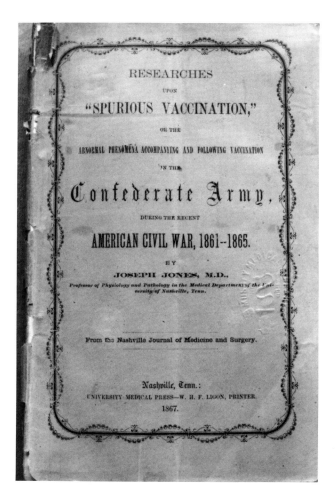

Postwar document (1867) that reported on the use of vaccination for small pox during the War of Rebellion.

Small pocket handbook that was presented to soldiers. It contains suggestions on ways to keep healthy. A few were: 1. Colored blankets are warmest. 2. Never lie down or sit down on the grass or bare earth for a moment. 3. Let the whole beard grow but not longer than three inches. 4. Flannel—wear it all over in all weather. 5. Bowels—The very moment you experience any uncomfortable sensation about the bowels, bind around them a piece of woolen cloth to support them and keep them warm. It also contains prayers and hymns.

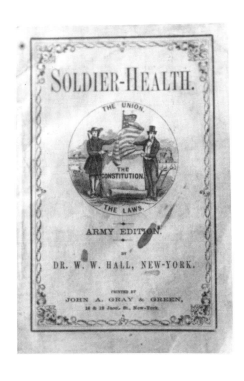

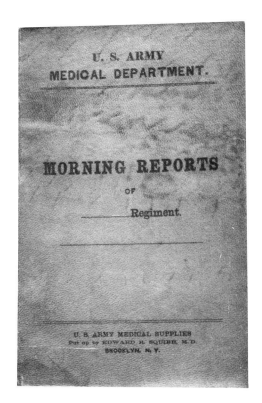

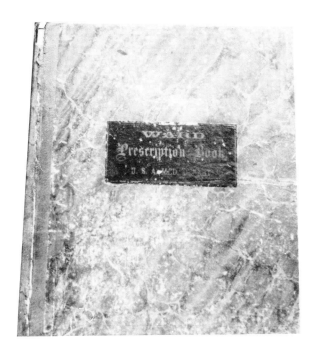

Regimental surgeons were to keep very accurate records of their soldiers' health. Edward Squibb, M.D., provided these morning report books so that this could be accomplished. It was also a vehicle for "advertising" Squibb Pharmaceutical Company.

Record-keeping book for the wards of hospitals. This book was kept by Surgeon Madell of the 20th New York Cavalry.

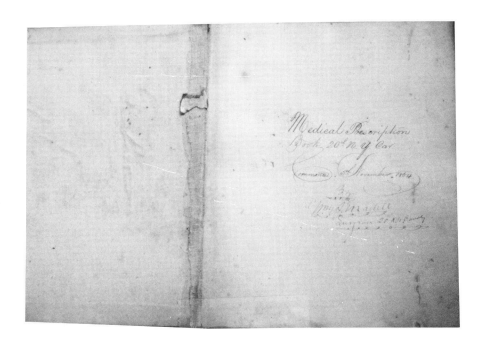

George M. Beakes.

NOTES ON THE SURGERY

OF THE

WAR IN THE CRIMEA,

WITH REMARKS ON

THE TREATMENT OF GUNSHOT WOUNDS.

BY

GEORGE H. B. MACLEOD, M.D., F.R.C.S.,

FORMERLY SURGEON TO THE CIVIL HOSPITAL AT SMYRNA, AND TO THE GENERAL HOSPITAL
IN CAMP BEFORE SEBASTOPOL;
LECTURER ON MILITARY SURGERY IN ANDERSON'S UNIVERSITY, GLASGOW, ETC.

PHILADELPHIA:
J. B. LIPPINCOTT & CO.
LONDON: JOHN CHURCHILL.
1862.

A source of knowledge for the Civil War surgeon was the experiences of the surgeon during the Crimean War. This book belonged to Surgeon George M. Beakes of the 1st New York Cavalry.

George M. Beakes
Cleuna House Hospital, Va.
1st New York Cav'g
Jan. 1862.

K.
Tin Sulpe ℥i
Fr. Ferri Chlorid. ℥ij
Aq. pur ℥iv
Coch proo. yr
nus — Typhoid.

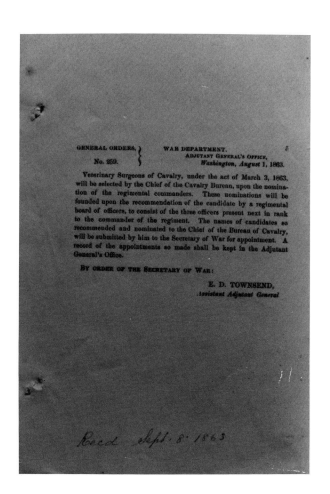

A very rare document that deals with the veterinary surgeon of the U.S. Cavalry. This very necessary branch of the Civil War army is often overlooked in historical accounts.

A relic of the medical office from the Confederate prison "Castle Thunder" in Richmond, Virginia. This was taken from the medical office door by a Union soldier when the prison was liberated in 1865.

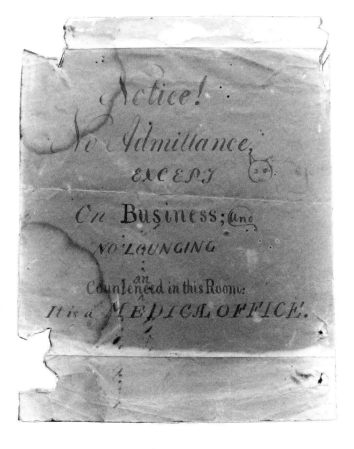

What Is It?

*M*any, many items are present that the author cannot find a use for. This last chapter will present these items, and perhaps a reader can help identify them.

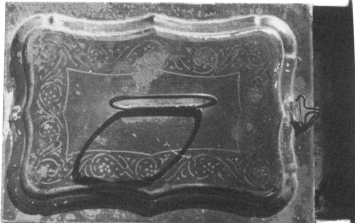

Tin carrying case with pull-out drawer. Marked *U.S. M. Dept.*. It is black in color with gold lettering and decorative stripping. The inside of the drawer has a hollow tube attached to it.

Top view.

Side view.

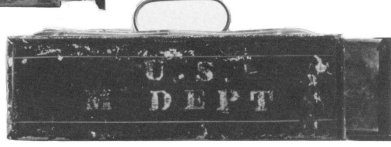

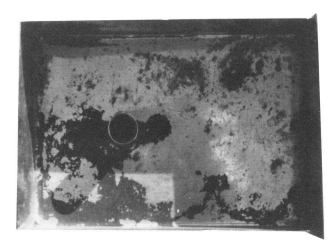

Top view of drawer.

Made entirely of hard rubber, this injection type device is *thought to be* an embalming instrument.

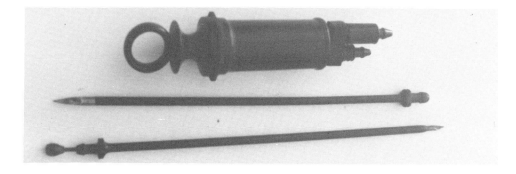

UNION SICKNESS

	Cases	Attack Rate	Deaths	Mortality Rate
Typhoid	75,368	2.6	27,050	35.9
Typhus	2,501	0.09	850	34.0
Continuous fever	11,898	0.4	147	1.2
Typho-malarial fever	49,871	1.7	4,059	8.1
Acute diarrhea	1,155,266	40.0	2,923	0.3
Chronic diarrhea	170,488	5.9	27,558	16.2
Acute dysentery	233,812	8.0	4,084	1.7
Chronic dysentery	25,670	0.9	3,229	12.6
Syphylis	73,382	2.5	123	0.2
Gonorrhea	95,833	3.3	6	0
Scurvy	30,714	1.1	383	1.2
Delerium tremens	3,744	0.1	450	12.0
Insanity	2,410	0.08	80	3.3
Paralysis	2,837	0.09	231	8.1
	1,933,794		71,173	3.7

UNION CAUSES OF DEATH

	Officers	Men	Total	Percent
Killed in action	4,142	62,916	67,058	18.7
Died of wounds	2,223	40,789	43,012	12.0
Died of disease	2,795	221,791	224,586	62.5
Accidental deaths	142	3,972	4,114	
Drowned	106	4,838	4,944	
Murdered	37	483	520	
Killed after capture	14	90	104	
Suicide	26	365	391	6.8
Executed by authorities	—	267	267	
Executed by enemy	4	60	64	
Sunstroke	5	308	313	
Other known causes	62	1,972	2,034	
Causes not stated	28	12,093	12,121	
	9,584	349,944	359,528	100

Courtesy of Mr. Dave Meyers and the "Society of Civil War Surgeons"

DEATHS

Union Enlistments	2,893,304
Deaths in Battle	110,070
Deaths from Disease	224,586
Accidents, Suicides, etc.	24,872
	359,528
	12.4%
Confederate Enlistments (Approx.)	1,317,035
Deaths in Battle	94,000
Deaths from Disease	164,000
	258,000
	19.6%

UNION WOUNDS

Gunshot	245,790	99.6%
Saber/Bayonet	992	0.4%
	246,712	100%

UNION MEDICAL CORPS

Surgeon General	Brigadier General	
Assistant Surgeon Gen.	Col.	
Medical Inspector Gen.	Col.	
Medical Inspector	Lt. Col.	16
Surgeon USA	Major	170
Assistant Surgeon USA	1st Lt. or Capt.	
Surgeon USV	Major	597
Assistant Surgeon USV	1st Lt.	
Regimental Surgeon		2109
Regimental Ass't Surgeon	State Comm	3882
Acting Staff Surgeon		85
Acting Assistant Surgeon	No Comm	5532
		12344

PHYSICIAN CASUALTIES

32	Killed in battle or by guerillas
9	Killed by accidents
	Wounded in action (83)
10	Died of wounds
4	Died in prison
7	Died of yellow fever
3	Died of cholera
271	Died of other diseases
336 =	2.7% Casualties
	5.0% Casualties in field service